# MECHANISMS OF
# NERVOUS DISORDER
## AN INTRODUCTION

# MECHANISMS OF
# NERVOUS DISORDER
## AN INTRODUCTION

### DAVID BOWSHER
MA, MD, PhD

Reader in the
Department of Anatomy,
University of Liverpool,
Honorary Consultant,
Department of Medical and
Surgical Neurology,
Walton Hospital, Liverpool

BLACKWELL SCIENTIFIC PUBLICATIONS
OXFORD LONDON EDINBURGH MELBOURNE

© 1978 Blackwell Scientific Publications
Osney Mead, Oxford OX2 oEL
8 John Street, London, WC1N 2ES
9 Forrest Road, Edinburgh EH1 2QH
P.O. Box 9, North Balwyn, Victoria, Australia

First published 1978

British Library Cataloguing in
Publication Data

Bowsher, David
    Mechanisms of nervous disorder.
    1. Nervous system – Diseases
    I. Title
    616.8         RC346

    ISBN 0–632–00075–9


Distributed in the USA by
J.B. Lippincott Company, Philadelphia
and in Canada by
J.B. Lippincott Company of Canada Ltd, Toronto


Printed in Great Britain by
Billing & Sons Limited,
Guildford, London and Worcester

# CONTENTS

# PREFACE

Many of my students have asked me to continue my *Introduction to the Anatomy and Physiology of the Nervous System* into the field of applied neurobiology which they encounter during their clinical studies. This companion volume is the result, and arises from my experience in teaching students during their clinical attachments; it attempts to show how neurological disorder in man can be understood on the basis of the anatomy and physiology of the nervous system.

My particular thanks are due to Mr C.B. Sedzimir, Director of Studies in Neurosurgery, and Head of the Associated Unit of Neurosciences, University of Liverpool, and to Dr L.A. Liversedge, Head of the Department of Neurology, University of Manchester, who have both read the text with great care, and offered helpful and constructive criticisms.

The illustrations have been specially prepared by Mr K.T. Briggs, to whom I wish to express my gratitude. Figures 2, 6, 7, 8, 9, 10 and 11 are based on outlines in *Structure of the Human Brain: A Photographic Atlas* by S.J. DeArmond, M.M. Fusco, and M.M. Dewey, published by Oxford University Press (New York); I am grateful to the authors and publishers for permission to use them. The index has been prepared by Mr F.W. Wallis, and the manuscript typed by Miss C. Whiting, to both of whom I express my thanks.

*Liverpool, March* 1977                    DAVID BOWSHER

# INTRODUCTION

This is not a textbook of neurology. It does not attempt to explain the aetiology, pathology, prognosis, or treatment of any neurological *disease*. Nor is it concerned with the order of appearance of symptoms and signs or their evolution over time, consideration of all which are of fundamental importance in arriving at the diagnosis of a particular disease.*

The purpose of this text is to explain, on a scientific basis, the whys and wherefores of neurological *disorder*. It attempts to show how the signs and symptoms which are met with in patients whose nervous system is damaged by disease or trauma can be accounted for in terms of interrupted connections or functions. The first step towards such clinical understanding is obviously to have some knowledge of the structure and function of the normal nervous system; the author's contribution to this aspect is embodied in his *Introduction to the Anatomy and Physiology of the Nervous System (IAPNS)*, to which reference is frequently made in the present text. But when the nervous system is damaged, the resulting disorder cannot in many instances be explained

* Throughout this text, reference is made to disease states which can be responsible for the abnormal functions described. It is therefore possible, by judicious use of the index, to find the majority of signs and symptoms which may occur in any given neurological disorder; but only by clinical encounter and through clinical teaching will it be possible to use this information to arrive at a diagnosis.

simply by subtracting the function subserved by the damaged part from the totality of known nervous function; it is also a question of understanding what system A will do when system B is not working.

Secondly, in addition to the consideration of what might be termed the lop-sided neurological function which occurs in disease or trauma, it is necessary to understand how such dysfunction finds its expression in our own sentient and communicating species. To take but one of many instances which will be encountered in the ensuing chapters, animal experiment has established that a minor partial lesion of the corticospinal pathway results in a particular type of motor deficit; but could never have told us that it causes the subjective impression of 'heaviness' in the affected limb. Furthermore, function is tested, and dysfunction demonstrated, in special ways in man because he can obey verbal commands and tell us what he feels.

Lastly, it is worth while to re-state the truism that abnormality of function can only be distinguished by comparison with the normal. It is therefore absolutely essential that students of medicine take every opportunity to test, and so to become familiar with, the normal by carrying out frequent neurological examinations on their peers by the methods which they are taught by their clinical instructors. Until one is thoroughly at home with the wide range of normal variation, and knows what it feels like to be examined (for half of it depends on what the patient says he feels), it will be impossible to detect objective or subjective variations from the normal.

# CHAPTER 1
# PERIPHERAL NERVES

Peripheral nerve fibres, both efferent from and afferent to the spinal cord and brainstem are functionally segregated according to fibre diameter (*IAPNS*, Chapter 4), though with some degree of overlap. This is of importance when considering disorders affecting peripheral nerves, for fibres are differentially susceptible to various forms of insult as a function of their size.

As a first example, local anaesthesia with procaine or a related compound may be considered—as in dental anaesthesia of the inferior dental nerve. It is common experience that such a procedure blocks pain sensation, while leaving a sense of touch-pressure. This is because the chemical first attacks small nerve fibres (groups C or IV and Aδ or III) which conduct impulses generated by noxious and thermal stimulation, while large fibres (group Aβ or II) coming from low-threshold mechanoreceptors are spared by the concentrations used in clinical practice. Similar results are produced, sometimes permanently, by substances such as phenol which can be manoeuvred onto dorsal roots within the subarachnoid space for the relief of pain in an appropriate root distribution.

Although in such cases the sense of touch may be preserved, tactile stimulation does not feel normal. This is because such natural stimuli as prodding with a finger normally excite receptors associated with afferent fibres of all sizes—in the case of touch-pressure more big ones than little ones, but some little ones all the same. If impulses are prevented from passing in the smaller fibres, the sensation evoked by tactile stimulation will arise from an unusual, abnormal pattern of impulses reaching the central nervous system, and so will 'feel funny'. Strictly speaking, such an abnormal sensation is referred to as a *paraesthesia*, though the term is more usually employed only for those abnormal sensations, apparently spontaneous, which are popularly called 'pins and needles', and which tend to occur when large fibres are selectively inactivated. Small nerve fibres are not often affected by disease in the absence of large fibre damage. The converse, however, is quite common, and may be illustrated by compressing the upper limb with a sphygmomanometer cuff. If a cuff around the arm is inflated to a pressure above systolic, sensation disappears in the order: touch-pressure, joint sensation, thermaesthesia, pinprick and (much later) deep pain. The explanation, in part at least, is that the nerve is rendered ischaemic. The largest nerve fibres, with the highest metabolic rate, are the first to be affected, while the smallest, with the lowest metabolic rate, are the last to be put out of action. This type of partial conduction block will occur whenever a nerve trunk or nerve root is compressed; an example of the former is cervical rib (or 'thoracic inlet syndrome') when the brachial plexus is stretched over bone.

Nerve root compression is illustrated by herniated intervertebral disc, when a lower lumbar or upper sacral root is stretched across the protrud'ng disc. Diabetic and other forms of peripheral neuropathy may also produce these dissociated sensory disorders. An arch example is post-herpetic neuralgia, in which the dorsal root ganglion cells of the large fibres are actually destroyed by the virus, perhaps in part due to compression when they try to swell within the unyielding fibrous capsule of the ganglion; the condition most commonly occurs in intercostal and first division trigeminal nerves.

Many of the conditions due to partial anoxia of peripheral sensory nerves with loss of sensory modalities carried by large fibres are accompanied by hyperalgesia or even 'spontaneous' pain. This is a complex subject, more fully dealt with in Chapter 7. In some cases where the compression is mechanical, such as herniated intervertebral disc, the unaffected small fibres may be depolarized, and thus activated, by the mechanical stimulus.

The preceding paragraphs are concerned with the general mechanisms of disordered physiology which may afflict peripheral sensory nerves. Some attention should be given to the anatomical factors which make possible the localization of peripheral nerve lesions. It should be possible to determine whether a lesion is in an individual nerve, a plexus, or a dorsal root, by correlating the distribution of sensory change with anatomy—remembering that it is not shameful to consult one of the large textbooks of general anatomy if necessary. One proviso must be entered: since some pathological processes affect long axons before short ones, organic disease may produce a seemingly unanatomical glove or stocking distribution of sensory change, in which the distal parts of limbs are affected; such distribution is therefore not necessarily a certain sign of purely functional or 'hysterical' disorder, as stated in some older textbooks, nor of a lesion in the appropriate region of the somatosensory cortex.

The $\alpha$-motor neurone and its peripheral axon are known clinically as the *lower motor neurone* (LMN); the cell body is situated in the somatic efferent or branchiomotor columns of cranial nerve nuclei or in the anterior horn (Rexed lamina IX) of the spinal grey matter. The LMN is the final common pathway from the central nervous system to the effector constituted by striated muscle. Destruction of the LMN obviously leads to a total loss of control by the central nervous system of the muscle concerned, and results in *flaccid paralysis*, in which there is total loss of tone, and of all voluntary and reflex movement in the muscle. Due to disease, the muscle rapidly wastes, and eventually becomes fibrosed unless steps are taken to prevent this.

The LMN can be affected at several points. Within the central nervous system, the cell body of the $\alpha$-motor neurone may be destroyed. A common such cause is the virus of poliomyelitis, although other forms of motor neurone disease (progressive muscular atrophy, chronic bulbar palsy) are encountered. There are also well-recognized pathological entities which affect both upper (see Chapter 2) and lower motor neurones.

Fibrillation or *fasciculation* of muscle, when present, is a pathognomonic sign of lower motor neurone involvement, usually in the region of the cell body; it never occurs when only upper motor neurones are affected. Peripherally, trauma is the most obvious cause of LMN lesions. Some forms of peripheral neuritis affect motor rather than sensory nerves. This is notably the case with lead poisoning, which, though a general neurotoxin, has a predilection for the distal portion of the radial nerve, leading to wrist drop. Ischaemia, the mechanism of which was mentioned in connection with sensory nerves, is concerned not with direction of conduction but only with fibre size; it may therefore affect motor nerves. Compression of roots (herniated intervertebral disc) or a nerve or plexus (e.g. cervical rib) can therefore produce signs of lower motor neurone disorder.

Although they can occur in the cervical region, the vast majority of herniated intervertebral discs are seen in either the L4–5 or L5–S1 interspaces. In the former the knee jerk (quadriceps tendon reflex) and the latter the ankle jerk (gastrocnemius-soleus tendon reflex) are diminished or lost. It is a moot point as to whether the reflex is affected because of ischaemia of the Ia fibres, afferent from muscle spindles and the largest of all peripheral axons, of the afferent arc, or because of ischaemia of the $\alpha$-motor neurone axons of the efferent arc, or both. It should be borne in mind that in cases of peripheral (motor) neuritis or nerve compression, the LMN lesion is frequently partial or subtotal, so that instead of complete flaccid paralysis and reflex loss, weakness and diminished reflexes are often found. Most forms of *peripheral neuritis* (neuropathy) affect both LMNs and primary afferents, so that the symptoms may include weakness, loss of tendon jerks, paraesthesia, diminution or loss of low-threshold mechanoreceptive sensation and muscular tenderness—the latter perhaps due to the action of unmyelinated muscle afferents in the absence of central inhibition brought about by activity in larger afferents. Visible fasciculation is rare in peripheral neuropathy.

The junction between a lower motor neurone and muscle (motor end plate) is a synapse, in which the excitatory transmitter substance is acetylcholine (ACh). Transmission at this synapse is blocked by curare and synthetic curarizing agents, which is why they are used as muscle relaxants in surgery. There is also a disease, myasthenia gravis, in which transmission from nerve to muscle is affected. Primary muscle diseases, usually with a heredo-familial background, also exist. In some of them, certain muscle groups may show pseudohypertrophy while others show only wasting. Unless disuse atrophy of the muscle is severe LMN dysfunction may be diagnosed by the fact that while electrical stimulation of the motor nerve produces no response, direct stimulation of the muscle still causes it to contract. This test may serve crudely to differentiate LMN disease from primary muscle diseases in which direct stimulation of muscle is less effective.

## THE CRANIAL NERVES

It is usual to examine the cranial nerves in more or less numerical order; some slight exceptions will be made in the descriptive order to be used in this chapter, in the interest of functional and anatomical tidiness. In general, patients as well as medical practitioners are more aware of the face (and hands) than of other parts of the body, so there is a tendency for disorders in this region to be noticed and reported at a somewhat earlier stage than if occurring elsewhere, although, as will be seen in Chapter 6, there are some remarkable exceptions.

The *olfactory nerve* is rarely affected by anything other than so-called olfactory groove meningioma or trauma in the region of the cribriform plate—the latter sometimes occurring by contre-coup as a result of a blow to the back of the head as a shearing injury. Frontal injury may be accompanied by dural tearing, resulting in cerebrospinal rhinorrhoea. The ability to smell should be tested separately in each nostril. Olfactory disorders other than total or partial loss of smell usually betoken a lesion in the temporal lobe of the forebrain.

## THE EYES AND THEIR SURROUNDINGS

More information about the nervous system can be gleaned by examination of the eyes and their immediate surroundings than by any other simple procedure. Such scrutiny will reveal disorders of the second, third, fourth, sixth and parts of the fifth and seventh cranial nerves, as well as of the superior cervical sympathetic ganglion.

The *upper eyelid* (levator palpebrae superioris) is made up mainly of striated muscle innervated by the somatic efferent component of the third (oculomotor) nerve, and partly of smooth muscle supplied by sympathetic fibres emanating from the superior cervical ganglion. Drooping of the eyelid (*ptosis*) therefore implies involvement of one or both of these. If the upper eyelid completely covers the eye, it is invariably the third nerve which is affected. In the case of an incomplete ptosis, it may be either the third nerve or the sympathetic which is involved, but the issue can usually be easily decided by examination of the pupil (*vide infra*). Primary muscular disorder, particularly myasthenia gravis, can also give rise to ptosis; since the levator palpebrae superioris is active during every waking moment, it is not surprisingly frequently the first muscle to be affected. Myasthenic ptosis, of course, tends to be bilateral, though not necessarily symmetrical. It should be noted that the converse disorder, an inability to cover the eye with the lids, such that incomplete closure (especially if unilateral) leaves part of the eyeball still visible to the observer, is a sign of dysfunction in the seventh nerve, which innervates the orbicularis oculi including the lower lid—for in eye closure, the lower lid moves as well as the upper.

*Pupillary size* should be equal on the two sides. Pupillary dilation is brought about by the sympathetic, and constriction by the visceral efferent component of the oculomotor nerve. The most noticeable disorder is a unilaterally constricted pupil due to the unopposed action of the third nerve pupilloconstrictors in the case of a lesion in the sympathetic fibres. In such a case, there may be other signs on the same side of the face due to failure of sympathetic action: since the sympathetically innervated sweat glands will not be working, the side of the face will have a dry smooth appearance. This symptom complex is known as Horner's syndrome, and is pathognomonic of a lesion of the sympathetic chain between the level of the first thoracic segment and the carotid bifurcation. Unilateral pupilloconstriction without concomitant changes in the facial skin can only occur if sympathetic fibres around the internal carotid or ophthalmic arteries are interrupted.

Unilateral pupillary dilation due to the unopposed action of the sympathetic implies a lesion of the parasympathetic efferent lower motor neurone in the oculomotor nerve. It is most often found in association with a concomitant lesion of the somatic efferent component of the third nerve, and of the fourth and sixth nerves as well, i.e. a paralysis of the external ocular muscles. This results in the 'fixed dilated pupil' of external ophthalmoplegia, and anatomical considerations make it evident that the three nerves can be affected together in the cavernous sinus (e.g. by venous thrombosis or internal carotid aneurysm), in the superior orbital fissure (e.g. by a meningioma), or within the orbit; in this last case, especially if the lesion is a tumour, there is frequently some degree of protrusion of the eyeball (proptosis).

It should be noted that the foregoing applies entirely to inspection of the resting pupil and is no way concerned with changes in the pupillary light reflexes, which would signify lesions of an arc whose afferents travel through the visual pathway to the midbrain.

*Ocular movements* are normally conjugate and are controlled peripherally by the third, fourth, and sixth nerves. Centrally, there are further bilateral controls on the nuclei of these nerves both by neurones originating in the cortex, and by the medial longitudinal fasciculus (Figs. 1 and 2) which interconnects the vestibular nuclei and the somatic efferent nuclei of the third, fourth and sixth nerves; in addition to the medial longitudinal fasciculus, connections between the vestibular nuclei and the lower motor neurones concerned with ocular movements are also effected through the reticular formation.

It is most important to bear in mind that the fundamental biological purpose of these intricate mechanisms (to which reflex turning of the head on the neck, effected by tectospinal pathways, may be added) is to keep the image of whatever is being looked at on the macula, and to achieve smooth fusion of the images on the two retinae. In general, then, it follows that unilateral failure of any particular ocular movement or movements signals a lower motor neurone lesion—and indeed in most cases an extracerebral lesion, while bilaterally symmetrical afflictions tend to be of central origin. Disorders of cortical and tectal origin are dealt with in Chapter 6.

The commonest, and most easily diagnosed, of the single nerve lesions is abducent palsy. In this condition, the eye on the affected side cannot be abducted beyond the midline; it presents because the patient complains of seeing double when looking to the affected side. Isolated loss of function in the fourth nerve is probably commoner than is thought for the

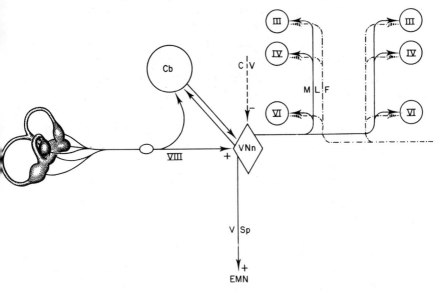

FIG. 1. Connections of the vestibular nuclei. Bipolar neurones of the vestibular division of the eighth nerve (VIII) convey excitatory (+) impulses from the vestibular apparatus to the vestibular nuclei (VNn); a few primary vestibular fibres pass directly to the cortex of the anterior lobe vermis, flocculus, and nodulus of the cerebellum (Cb). These parts of the cerebellum also receive secondary vestibular afferents from the vestibular nuclei; and they, together with the fastigial nucleus, project to the vestibular nuclei. The dotted line (CV) indicates the tonic inhibitory (-) input to the vestibular nuclei from the cerebral cortex, probably relayed through the interstitial nucleus of Cajal in the midbrain.

Efferent fibres from the vestibular nuclei are in two main groups: (i) the vestibulospinal tract (VSp), arising mainly in the lateral vestibular nucleus of Deiters, has a facilitatory effect (+) on lower limb antigravity extensor motorneurones (EMN); (ii) The medial longitudinal fasciculus (MLF) arises chiefly from the superior and medial vestibular nuclei, and projects to the abducent (VI), trochlear (IV), and oculomotor (III) nuclei of both sides as well as to the interstitial nucleus of Cajal and the nucleus of Darkschewitsch (not shown) in the midbrain just rostral to the third nerve nucleus.

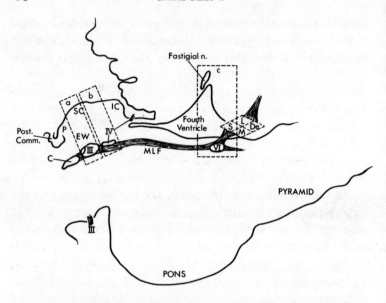

FIG. 2.   Schematic parasagittal section of the brainstem, to show the
medial longitudinal fasciculus (MLF) and its connections.

Post. Comm. = Posterior Commissure, above which is the pineal gland
(not shown)

C = Interstitial nucleus of Cajal, probably the relay for descending
inhibitory influences on the lateral vestibular nucleus (L).

P = Pretectal region; receives direct afferent connections from the
retina and projects indirectly to the Edinger–Westphal (EW) nucleus
of the oculomotor nucleus (III). This region is the 'centre' for the light
and accommodation reflexes. Superior (SC) and inferior (IC) colliculi.
Note their topographical relationship to the oculomotor (III) and
trochlear (IV) nuclei.

S,L,M, De = Superior, Lateral (Deiters'), Medial, and Descending
vestibular nuclei. They are shown in dotted outline because they are in
fact far lateral to the plane of the rest of the diagram. Vestibular nuclear
efferents to the MLF come chiefly from the superior and medial
nuclei. MLF afferents, probably from the interstitial nucleus of Cajal
(C) end mainly in the lateral nucleus.

Lesions in plane a will chiefly affect upward gaze.

Lesions in plane b will chiefly affect downward gaze.

Lesions in plane c (which includes the cerebellar vermis, fastigial
nucleus, part of the superior vestibular nucleus, and abducent nucleus
(VI)) will chiefly affect lateral gaze.

simple reasons that of itself many patients would not notice it and would not therefore report it; and that if it occurs in association with other non-ophthalmoplegic signs, it may be overlooked in the course of a neurological examination. Since the superior oblique muscle, innervated by the trochlear nerve, causes the ocular globe to turn downwards and outwards, there will be a diplopia for objects to see which the affected eye would have to rotate in this direction—for example, when trying to read a book held in the hand of the affected side.

All the extrinsic muscles except the lateral rectus and the superior oblique, but including the striated component of the upper eyelid, are supplied by the somatic efferent component of the third nerve. Ptosis has already been mentioned and is probably the most frequently-occurring form of isolated partial third nerve lesion. However, it is not uncommon to find other muscles innervated by the third nerve affected singly. There appears to be no anatomical rhyme or reason for loss of function in single muscles, or the order in which it appears in progressive cases. Sometimes, however, there is clearly an affection of the superior ramus (innervating the levator palpebrae superioris and superior rectus muscle) or the inferior ramus, which supplies the other orbital muscles (medial and inferior recti, inferior oblique) and also

---

The exact site and nature of the lesion determines whether it will be characterized by nystagmus or a paralysis of gaze.

Lesions in the vestibular nerve (VIIIv) or nuclei as a whole, if affecting input from all three semicircular canals, tend to cause rotatory nystagmus.

Disorders of lateral gaze can also result from lesions in the frontal and occipital eye fields (not shown). Man, like most other earthbound (as opposed to aquatic, arboreal or aerial) creatures, is chiefly concerned with movements in the horizontal plane—whether those movements be his own or those of external objects. For this biological reason, disorders (paralysis, nystagmus) of horizontal (lateral) gaze are very much more common than disorders of vertical gaze.

carries the parasympathetic fibres which pass to the ciliary ganglion; this is most likely to occur when the lesion is peripheral to the superior orbital fissure.

When lesions of the fourth, sixth or branches of the third nerve occur, the optic axes fail to keep parallel when turning in a direction which would involve using the functionally-denervated muscles, thus giving rise to diplopia when looking in the appropriate direction; it is often 'seeing double' in part of the visual field of which the patient complains. It may sometimes be noticed that the head is held in an unusual position so as to avoid diplopia; this in its turn may give rise to dizziness, due to failure to 'balance up' the information coming from the two vestibular organs. When a lesion of the third nerve is suspected, testing accommodation and the direct and consensual reaction to illumination may reveal unilateral loss of function in the constrictor pupillae; if (unilaterally) positive, it is a clear lower motor neurone lesion in the third nerve. It should be noted that in some cases, usually of nuclear lesions in the midbrain, either some or all of the striated muscles of the eyeball or the constrictor pupillae are paralysed on one side.

Separate extracerebral lower motor neurone lesions of the nerves to the extraocular muscles are seen apart from causes already mentioned essentially in two sets of circumstances. In the first, there is direct involvement of parts or all of the third nerve and/or the whole of the sixth nerves due to disease process in the meninges to which they are intimately related. Such conditions include lesions in the cavernous sinus, (localized) acute or chronic meningitis and meningioma, and in such cases the resulting ocular palsies may prove a valuable localizing sign. Subarachnoid haemorrhage too, especially when originating from an aneurysm of the internal carotid or adjacent posterior communicating artery, may involve the nerves on the affected side due to the close anatomical relationship. In the second group, ocular palsies may occur due to stretching or compression of nerves caused by space-occupying lesions (Chapter 5). In such instances (which include many cases of subarachnoid haemorrhage), only third nerve lesions have any value as a localizing sign.

*Nystagmus* is a slow repetitive conjugate deviation of the eyes away from the line of optic fixation, followed by a quick return; it most often occurs only when the eyes are turned in a particular direction. Although nystagmus is conventionally described in terms of the direction of the rapid component, it must be thoroughly understood that it is the slow deviation from the direction of gaze which is abnormal, not the rapid return to it. In order to understand the mechanism of nystagmus, every student should see and experience the effect of inducing nystagmus by irrigating the external auditory meatus while lying on the side with water at 44°C and at 30°C. In both cases, convection currents are set up in the vestibular semi-circular canals, particularly the horizontal canal—so that the resulting nystagmus is chiefly horizontal. Warm water provokes an outward (upward when laterally horizontal) deviation of the cupola and nystagmus with its slow component towards the irrigated side; cold water an inward (downward when laterally horizontal) deviation and nystagmus with its slow component away from the irrigated side. Correlation with the anatomy of the vestibular apparatus shows that the (slow) ocular deviation is in the same direction as the movement of the cupola. Thus, for example, in the normal, when the head is turned to the right, the rotational acceleration in the horizontal canals swings the cupola to the right and the gaze follows, under the influence of vestibularly-generated excitation in the medial longitudinal fasciculus (Fig. 1). When the cupolae are made to deviate artificially, without head turning, the eyes are fooled into turning (slowly) in the same direction, but then rapidly return; hence nystagmus.

It is equally evident from the foregoing that what the medial longitudinal fasciculus does is (1) to co-ordinate the activities of the motor nuclei controlling the extra-ocular muscles so as to produce conjugate movements of the eyes, and (2) to subserve vestibulo-ocular reflexes. Anatomically, it will be recalled (Figs. 7, 9, and 10), the medial longitudinal fasciculi of the two sides closely embrace the nuclei of the third, fourth and sixth nerves, so that a destructive lesion of one of the latter is liable to involve the adjacent fasciculus, or vice versa. The paralysis of gaze which results, happily for the factually-overburdened student, can be related to the function of the appropriate nucleus (Fig. 2). Thus for example, a lesion in the region of the right abducent nucleus would produce deficiency of conjugate deviation to the right, while a lesion in the midbrain tends to produce paralyses of upward and/or downward gaze.

Pathological nystagmus may be of peripheral origin, when the disease process is in the vestibular organ or nerve, or of central origin, due to pathology of the vestibular nuclei or their afferent and efferent connections. Since disease of the sense organ as in labyrinthitis or Menière's syndrome usually affects the input from all three semicircular canals, the nystagmus is often rotatory or semi-rotatory, i.e. with a rotatory slow component and a horizontal quick return. For the same reason, this type of nystagmus is also seen in disease of the vestibular nerve. The commonest such affection to come to neurological attention is eighth nerve sheath tumour, which will also produce disorders of the acoustic division of the nerve (deafness, sometimes associated with tinnitus) and signs of compression of structures in the posterior fossa (Chapter 4). Vertigo or dizziness is an invariable concomitant of any process, peripheral or central, which interferes with the neural input from the vestibular apparatus, perhaps because of the failure of the central nervous system to match up the normal input from one side with the abnormal input from the other. It is generally taught that vestibular vertigo makes the subject feel as though he/she is rotating towards the side of the lesion, as opposed to cerebellar vertigo in which external objects appear to rotate away from the side of the lesion. On examination, however, real living patients are hardly ever as definite as this. More is to be gained by asking the subject to describe the direction of rotation during an attack: a patient with, e.g. a right-sided vestibular lesion will say 'Either I am rotating clockwise or the room is rotating anticlockwise', while the patient with a right-sided medial cerebellar lesion will say 'Either the room or myself is rotating anticlockwise'. In other words, in vestibular vertigo the sense of subjective rotation is in the opposite direction to that of the apparent rotation of external objects, whereas in cerebellar vertigo they are both in the same direction. However, when the disease process (or its therapy) result in cessation of input from the affected side, compensation is fairly rapidly made (over a few weeks) so the nystagmus and vertigo may disappear.

Central lesions in the brainstem causing nystagmus are most frequently due to multiple sclerosis. Since this protean disease is multifocal, and commonly involves the cerebellum as well, it is often difficult to localize the lesion(s) in the absence of other signs. However, nystagmus of brainstem origin is rarely rotatory, and is usually persistent. Lesions in the lower brainstem, between the vestibular and abducent nuclei, are said to give rise to horizontal nystagmus and midbrain lesions to vertical, thus corresponding in direction with the paralyses of gaze which ensue from lesions in the same areas.

The midline cerebellum, in the form of the anterior lobe vermis, projecting to the fastigial nuclei, as well as the flocculo-nodular lobe, have profuse twoway connections with the vestibular nuclei (Fig. 1), and thence with both the medial longitudinal fasciculus and the vestibulospinal upper motor neurone (Chapter 2). It is therefore not surprising that some cerebellar lesions affect eye movements; this will be dealt with in Chapter 4.

Although the division is not physiologically absolute, it can be said in general terms that the semicircular canals of the vestibular apparatus, which are excited by angular acceleration, influence eye movements, while the otolithic vestibular apparatus (utriculus and sacculus), sensitive to gravity, head position, and linear acceleration, influence the somatic musculature through the vestibulospinal upper motor neurone (Chapter 2).

What has been said about eye movements in this section depends on mechanisms in four cranial nerve nuclei (III, IV, VI, and VIII vestibular) and the connections between them (medial longitudinal fasciculus). Eye movements and pupillary reactions may also be influenced by interconnections between the cerebral cortex and reflex centres in the midbrain; this will be dealt with in Chapter 6, since disorders of this type have their main importance in the localization of supratentorial lesions.

The *second cranial nerve* is, of course, not properly speaking a peripheral nerve at all, but a central fibre pathway analogous to the medial lemniscus. The term optic nerve is applied to the part of the retino-geniculo-tectal tract between the eye and the optic chiasma, and it is with this part of the visual pathway only that this section will be concerned. It must always be borne in mind that afferent fibres in the optic nerve are responsible not only for conscious sensation of vision, but also for the unconscious pupillary reflexes. Some pathological conditions can dissociate these functions, and will be referred to in Chapter 6.

The optic fundus can be examined with the ophthalmoscope. It is absolutely essential that every medical student should learn to wield this instrument at the earliest opportunity, and become familiar with the normal appearance; this can and should be done by examining it through the pharmacologically dilated pupil of one's colleagues until such a degree of expertise is attained that dilatation is no longer necessary. Ophthalmoscopic examination is of great diagnostic importance in a number of systemic diseases, such as diabetes, hypertension, renal and arterial disease, as well as in ophthalmology and neurology, although it is only with the last-named that this section is concerned.

*Primary optic atrophy* is the sign of a dead optic nerve; because the nerve is dead, the optic disc becomes pearly white, and its margin with the surrounding pink retina appears particularly clear-cut. Symptomatically, of course, it is associated with failure of vision leading to blindness. Primary optic atrophy may be caused by any lesion which compresses (e.g. tumour, aneurysm) or damages (e.g. cranial trauma) the optic nerve, or by some forms of chemical poisoning. *Papilloedema* is swelling of the optic nerve head and its leading feature is filling of the optic cup, so that the disc becomes level with or even bulges forward out from the rest of the retina instead of being in a deeper plane. Such swelling obviously causes blurring of the edges of the optic disc, and this too is an important visible indication of papilloedema. In later stages, exudates and haemorrhages may be detected in the retina, due to obstruction of the venous return. Bilateral papilloedema is usually a sign of an increase in volume of the intracranial contents (space-occupying lesion, see Chapter 5), although the degree of papilloedema on the two sides may be unequal. Unilateral papilloedema may also be due to a space-occupying lesion, or to a local cause such as thrombosis of the central vein of the retina. While papilloedema sooner or later causes blurring of vision, the relationship between the two is most inconstant, and sometimes gross papilloedema is accompanied by very little blurring. A more constant sign, if carefully searched for, is enlargement of the blind spot of the retina. The normal blind spot is of course due to the absence of photoreceptors over the head of the optic nerve; in papilloedema, exudation covers the photoreceptors surrounding the disc, leading to an enlargement of the non-photosensitive area of retina. If papilloedema is allowed to progress to *secondary atrophy* of the optic nerve, vision is irreversibly lost. Secondary optic atrophy, like primary, is also marked by a dead white disc; but can be distinguished from it by the fact that exudate fills the optic cup and blurs the disc margins and sometimes buries short lengths of the vessels, so that they may appear discontinuous.

Acute *retrobulbar neuritis* is another condition which leads to blurring of vision. It is most commonly caused by multiple sclerosis (of which it is not infrequently the first manifestation), and if the lesion is close to the nerve head may be accompanied by swelling and oedema of the optic disc. As in the early stages of primary optic atrophy, the visual field(s) may exhibit a central scotoma. However, in cases due to multiple sclerosis, the visual symptoms usually disappear quite rapidly, but evidence of the condition remains as pallor of the temporal half of the optic disc.

The *corneal reflex* is afferently dependent on mechano-receptive fibres in the first division of the trigeminal nerve. While it can be elicited by touching the cornea with a wisp of cotton wool, the reflex is constantly in action and is necessary to keep the cornea evenly moistened and to sweep foreign particles towards the naso-lacrymal duct. The corneal reflex should be differentiated from the blink reflex, whose afferents are in the optic nerve and which operates when the eye is threatened.

One of the commonest causes of loss of corneal reflex is iatrogenic, due to interruption of the nerve (or its ganglion) for the treatment of trigeminal neuralgia. Loss of the reflex is a sign of corneal anaesthesia, and obviously may occur in any lesion involving the whole fifth nerve or its ophthalmic division. The corneal reflex should always be tested, because its loss can lead to the serious condition of corneal ulceration.

Both the corneal and blink reflexes are bilateral even though the provoking stimulus be unilateral. The efferent fibres of the reflex are in both cases in the seventh nerve, the active muscle being the orbicularis oculi, and not the levator palpebrae superioris. Loss of the blink reflex can therefore occur as a result of a seventh nerve lesion. Another ocular disorder which may occasionally be seen as a result of a seventh nerve lesion is *dry eye* due to interruption of the autonomic efferent fibres in the nervus intermedius which are preganglionic to the lacrymal glands. Paradoxical lachrymation will be referred to below.

## THE TRIGEMINAL NERVE

The motor root of the trigeminal nerve, forming part of the mandibular division, supplies the muscles of mastication, while each of the three afferent divisions is responsible for somatic sensation in a well-circumscribed area, with little overlap between branches. Since the trigeminal sensory nuclei are the only representatives of the somatic afferent column in the brainstem, it follows that all somatosensory fibres in the head region (e.g. those in the VIIth, IXth and Xth nerves) terminate in these nuclei. The distribution of any sensory disturbance, therefore, should be carefully mapped out, for it frequently enables the examiner to determine whether it is of peripheral or central origin; the latter may be seen at nuclear level in thrombosis of the posterior inferior cerebellar artery and in some cases of syringobulbia. Idiopathic trigeminal neuralgia however (Chapter 7), although believed by many to be of central origin, strictly respects the peripheral distribution of the affected division(s) of the trigeminal nerve; it is never associated with objective sensory loss.

Individual divisions or branches of the trigeminal nerve may be wholly or partly put out of action by infection by herpes zoster (see Chapter 7), trauma or space-occupying lesions. It is worth mentioning in this context that the ophthalmic division may be involved by an aneurysm of the internal carotid artery in the cavernous sinus, in which case loss of the corneal reflex will be observed; the periorbital and retrobulbar pain which is so typical of the condition has been attributed to irritation of the ophthalmic and maxillary nerves, but this explanation is not very satisfactory;* some authors have suggested that autonomic afferents in the wall of the internal carotid artery (and its branches) may be involved.

The whole nerve may be involved by cerebello-pontine angle tumours, of which by far the commonest is a sheath tumour of the eighth nerve, in which case other cranial nerves will also be affected. Tumours of this type on rare occasions arise from the sheath of the trigeminal nerve itself. Any lesion of the whole nerve at its exit from the pons, or to the mandibular division at any level within the skull will cause a lower motor neurone lesion of the muscles of mastication. Thanks to the synostosis between the two sides of the mandible a unilateral lesion may go almost unnoticed unless the examiner feels the temporal and masseter muscles when the jaw is clenched. However, it may be noted that when the mouth is actively opened (especially when this is done against resistance), the jaw is protruded towards the side of the lesion, due to the unopposed action of the lateral pterygoid muscle on the unparalysed side.

## THE SEVENTH NERVE

The intermediofacial nerve most obviously provides the motor innervation of the mimetic muscles; but it must be remembered that it also carries a visceral efferent component controlling the mucous glands of the nasal cavity as well as the lacrymal, submaxillary, and sublingual glands, a special afferent component responsible for gustatory sensation in the anterior two thirds of the tongue, and somatic afferent fibres for part of the external ear.

Isolated lesions of the seventh nerve are much commoner than those of the fifth. Careful attention to anatomy will

* Venous engorgement of the orbit resulting in proptosis and/or irritation of pericarotid sympathetic fibres, giving rise to a localized causalgia-like syndrome, are both more acceptable explanations.

confirm whether the lesion is proximal to the point at which the seventh nerve is joined by the chorda tympani, in which case taste will be affected, or distal, in which case it will not. A subtler point is the occurrence (or not) of hyperacusis auris, which can only happen if the nerve is damaged proximal to the point of departure of the nerve to stapedius.

These considerations apart, the signs of a lower motor neurone lesion in the seventh nerve are those of facial palsy, in which all the mimetic muscles are paralysed, including buccinator, so that the patient cannot blow, whistle or suck, and chews on the sound side in order to avoid the accumulation of food in the cheek. This is to be contrasted with an upper motor neurone lesion of the seventh nerve, in which there are two striking differences: (i) the forehead is not affected because it is represented in the cortex of both hemispheres; and (ii) emotional movements of the face may occur, even though voluntary movements below the level of the eyebrows are impaired.

Old lower motor neurone seventh nerve lesions, if no regeneration occurs, are frequently characterized by contractures in the facial muscles. This results in drawing up of the corner of the mouth on the affected side, so that, at a first glance, the impression is gained that the unaffected side is abnormal; the matter is easily settled by testing.

When regeneration occurs, the seventh nerve seems to show a particularly strong tendency for some sprouting axons to grow into the 'wrong' sheaths. There are two common consequences of this, one involving somatic (branchio-motor) efferent fibres, the other visceral (autonomic) efferents. The first involves mass action of the facial muscles, so that an attempt at an individual movement is converted into a grimace of the whole affected side of the face; the second often results in eating being accompanied by lacrymation as well as salivation.

Involvement of the *acoustic division of the eighth nerve* in disease process is characterized by tinnitus or deafness.

The *ninth, tenth and eleventh nerves* are most frequently injured unilaterally at their point of exit from the skull. Shoulder drop, or in incomplete lesions, inability to shrug the affected shoulder, due to total or partial paralysis of the trapezius, and loss of power in sternomastoid, make accessory nerve dysfunction easy to spot. Unilateral lesions of the ninth and tenth nerves, although affecting gustatory and somatic sensation on the posterior third of the tongue, and producing rapidly-compensated hoarseness, may go unnoticed; but the perspicacious examiner may observe asymmetry of palatal movements. Sheath tumours occasionally affect the glossopharyngeal nerve. Bilateral vagal palsy of supranuclear origin (see Chapter 4) is often fatal, due to respiratory obstruction.

The *hypoglossal nerve* may be damaged unilaterally or bilaterally in the brainstem by conditions such as syringobulbia, or peripherally in its canal, giving rise to a typical lower motor neurone paralysis of the tongue. Fasciculation is particularly easily seen; and on protrusion, the tongue deviates to the side of the lesion due to the unopposed action of the unaffected genioglossus muscle.

# CHAPTER 2
# CENTRAL MOTOR SYSTEMS

Central motor systems are several in number (*IAPNS*, Chapter 13), only one of which, the corticobulbospinal or pyramidal, runs without synapse from the cerebral cortex to the spinal cord. The other motor systems of clinical importance, corticorubrospinal, vestibulospinal, and so-called 'extrapyramidal' (Fig. 3) are trans-synaptically controlled from the cortex and/or the basal ganglia. The majority of long descending motor axons, with the important exception of corticospinal fibres controlling movement of the digits, do not synapse directly with lower motor neurones, but with segmental interneurones in the spinal grey matter (*IAPNS*, Fig. 19).

Two of the systems are somatotopically organized throughout; they are the functionally-interlinked corticobulbospinal system arising from cells in the fifth layer of the principal motor cortex (MI: area 4) of the precentral gyrus, and the corticorubrospinal, controlled from the supplementary motor cortex (part of area 6) on the medial surface of the hemisphere. For practical purposes, they may be said to exert their chief influence on distal and proximal limb muscles respectively. The vestibulospinal system is anatomically somatotopic, but in practical terms works as a whole; it receives tonic inhibitory control indirectly from the cortex, through a relay (interstitial nucleus of Cajal) in the upper midbrain (Fig. 2). The basal ganglia receive an input from

23

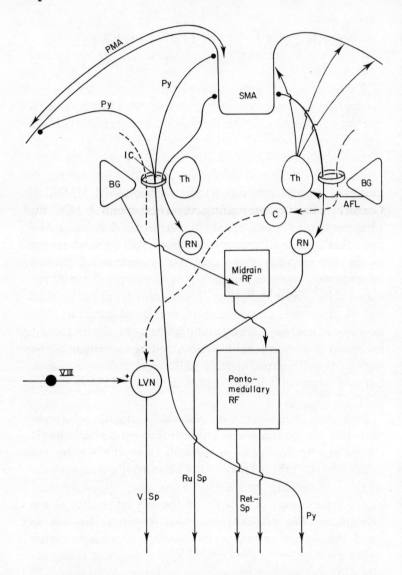

FIG. 3. Diagram to illustrate central motor systems and upper motor neurones

1. Fibres of the pyramidal tract (Py) arise from the cortex of the principal motor area (PMA) and pass through the internal capsule (IC)

many areas of the cortex and project polysynaptically onto pontine and medullary reticulospinal neurones; the whole of this system is incorrectly but traditionally called extra-pyramidal.

By definition, an *upper motor neurone* (*UMN*) *is the lowermost of the long descending neurones of a central motor system*; those of clinical importance being corticospinal (pyramidal), rubro-spinal, vestibulospinal, and reticulospinal (Fig. 3), the last-named being an UMN of the 'extrapyramidal' system. It may be noted immediately that, in anatomical terms, the internal capsule contains (i) the cortico-spinal UMN, (ii) cortical efferents controlling the rubrospinal UMN, and (iii) cortical efferents controlling the vestibulospinal UMN; but that it does *not* contain all the cortical fibres concerned with the 'extrapyramidal' system, because many of these

to reach LMN's (or their associated interneurones) in the contralateral cranial and spinal motor nuclei.

2. Fibres from the supplementary motor area (SMA) project through the internal capsule to the region of the red nucleus (RN), whence the crossed rubrospinal (RuSP) upper motorneurone passes down to influence chiefly those LMN's which innervate proximal limb muslces.

3. Cortical efferents (dashed lines) pass through the internal capsule to the interstitial nucleus of Cajal (C) in the upper midbrain, whence a further relay exerts a tonic inhibitory influence ( $-$ ) on the contra-lateral vestibular nucleus (LVN). The lateral vestibular nucleus, which is excited ( $+$ ) by sensory input through the vestibular nerve (VIII), gives rise to the uncrossed vestibulospinal (VSp) UMN, which has a facilitatory influence on lower limb extensor LMN's.

4. The complex 'extrapyramidal system' partly bypasses the internal capsule. Cortical efferents (not shown) pass to the basal ganglia (BG), which project to the descending midbrain reticular formation (RF). A further relay passes to the ponto-medullary reticular formation; and the UMN of the system may be regarded as the reticulospinal (Ret-Sp) fibres which influence the activity of LMN's.

However, the basal ganglia also project via the ansa and fasciculus lenticularis (AFL) to the thalamus (Th) and thence back to the principal and supplementary motor cortices; so that 'extrapyramidal' activity, both normal and abnormal, reaches LMN's through the systems des-cribed in 1, 2 and 3 above, as well as through the reticulospinal UMN.

relay in the basal ganglia and so manage to influence lower centres without passing through the internal capsule. However, direct cortical efferents to 'extrapyramidal' centres below the corpus striatum pass through the internal capsule.

A pure lesion of any upper motor neurone is characterized by:

(a)   Motor.deficit, tending to affect movements rather than muscles; it may be expressed by —plegia, paresis, difficulty in movement, or weakness.

(b)   Persistence of monosynaptic reflex activity (though this may be changed) in affected muscles because the lower motor neurone and its associated spinal (segmental) reflex arcs are intact.

(c)   Lack of wasting in the affected muscles, for the same reason, though some wasting through disuse may of course occur in the long term in untreated cases.

(d)   Changes in tone in the affected limbs, due to loss of descending influences on lower motor neurones.

## TONE IN UMN DISORDERS (Fig. 4)

The changes in tone which are observed in long-standing disorders of central motor systems (but not of the cerebellum) are virtually always in the direction of increase or hypertonus. By a hallowed tradition, this hypertonus is called 'spasticity' or 'rigidity' according to the type of disorder in which it is exhibited. These names however do not relate to the pathophysiology of hypertonus, of which three varieties may be recognized:

(i)   The corticospinal and rubrospinal tracts may be regarded as having a tonic inhibitory effect on phasic $\gamma$-motor neurones, which mostly innervate nuclear-bag intrafusal muscle fibres. When the descending inhibition is removed, there is no change in the tone of the affected muscle at rest. But as soon as the muscle is stretched (lengthened), exaggerated phasic stretch reflexes come into action, so that both abnormal resistance to stretch and exaggerated tendon jerks are observed. It should be added that the pyramidal tract also has an inhibitory action on extensor $\alpha$-motor neurones. In the case therefore of a corticospinal lesion, removal of this inhibition contributes to the hyper-reflexia which is most evident in extensors such as the quadriceps femoris and gastrocnemiussoleus. Their tendon reflexes may become exaggerated to such an extent as to become repetitively self-sustaining; a condition known as *clonus*.

(ii) Those reticulospinal upper motor neurones which become inactive in Parkinson's disease appear normally to have a tonic inhibitory action on the tonic (static) $\gamma$-motor neurones which mainly innervate nuclear-chain intrafusal muscle fibres. Removal of this descending inhibition therefore causes an increase in the resting tone of the affected muscles, but does not produce exaggeration of the tendon reflexes; this is the classical 'rigidity' of extrapyramidal disease.

(iii) Vestibulo-spinal upper motor neurones in man are normally facilitatory to the $\alpha$-motorneurones which control the extensor (antigravity) muscles of the ipsilateral lower limb. If the tonic descending inhibition which is normally exerted on the lateral vestibular nucleus is removed, extensor hypertonus of the lower limbs results.

It will have been noted that the first two types of hyper-tonus described above are reflex in nature. This can be demonstrated in patients suffering from the conditions which produce them, for infiltration of the muscle with a local anaesthetic solution which inactivates $\gamma$ efferents will abolish hypertonus; dorsal rhizotomy has been performed in the past for the (successful) abolition of pyramidal spasticity. It is highly significant in this context that in two disease entities—subacute combined degeneration and Friedreich's ataxia—in which there may occur simultaneous degeneration both of fibres in the lateral funiculus of the spinal cord, containing the pyramidal tract, and of the large primary afferents (including, for a short part of their course,

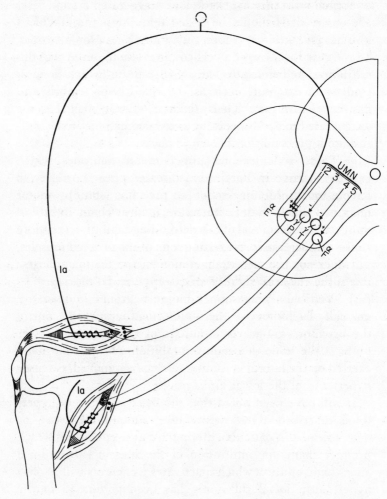

FIG. 4. Control of muscle tone. $a$-E and $a$-F are $a$-motorneurones supplying extensor and flexor extrafusal muscle fibres respectively. The extensor $a$-motorneurone is excited by the Ia spindle afferent from intrafusal fibres in its own muscle. In this diagram, the intrafusal fibre in the extensor muscle is illustrated as being supplied by a phasic $\gamma$-motorneurone ($\gamma$ −P), while the intrafusal fibre in the flexor muscle is shown as being supplied by a tonic $\gamma$-motorneurone ($\gamma$ −T).

$a$ − E is facilitated ($+$) not only by its own Ia spindle afferent, but those from muscle spindles) in the dorsal columns, flaccidity and loss of tendon reflexes are found rather than increase in tone and reflex activity; extensor plantar responses will however still be present. Vestibulospinal hypertonus, on the other hand, is (virtually) unaffected by inactivation of muscle afferents.

The *motor cortex* may be defined as that part of the neocortex which receives a point-to-point projection from the ventrolateral and ventroanterior thalamic nuclei (*IAPNS*, Chapter 12), and thus eventually feeds on information about the state of tension of muscles. Within this general area are two representations of the body. The principal motor area is roughly equivalent to the precentral gyrus, with the upsidedown representation such that the lower limb lies on the medial wall of the hemisphere in the territory of the anterior cerebral artery; the rest of the demihomunculus (or demimulieruncula) lies in the territory of the middle cerebral artery. The whole representation is inversely proportional to the size of motor units (*IAPNS*, Chapter 5), so that the

---

also by the vestibulospinal (1) upper motor neurone (UMN), while the pyramidal (2) pathway inhibits ( −) it tonically. Corticospinal and corticocorubrospinal UMNs also exert tonic inhibition on phasic $\gamma$-motorneurones (3) and facilitate flexor $\alpha$-motorneurones (5). Thus inactivation of corticospinal and corticorubrospinal (2, 3, 5) UMNs brings about (a) an increase in tendon jerks, particularly in extensor muscles, and (b) reflexly-activated spasticity which comes into action only when a muscle is passively elongated.

Inactivation of the vestibulospinal (1) UMN will lead to collapse of tone in antigravity muscles; while disinhibition of the vestibulospinal UMN (see Fig. 1) will cause a great increase in the tone of antigravity muscles, due to direct action of $\alpha$-motorneurones, and therefore not depending on the reflex mechanism operating through the spindle afferents.

The UMN (4) supplying tonic inhibition to tonic $\gamma$-motorneurones ($\gamma$ −T) is believed to be inactivated in some cases of 'extrapyramidal' disease, particularly paralysis agitans. Such a functional lesion would lead to a reflexly-maintained increase in resting tone ('rigidity'), but no increase in tendon jerks.

area of cortex devoted to digits, lips and tongue is relatively very large. The corticobulbospinal tract arises from cells in the fifth cortical layer in the principal motor area.

The supplementary motor area lies on the medial surface of the hemisphere (in part of Brodmann's area 6), in front of and below the lower limb area of the principal motor representation, above (dorsal to) the cingulate gyrus. In it, the body is represented lying with the head forward (rostrally, anteriorly), the back down towards the corpus callosum, and so the limbs up towards the vertex. There is much less exaggeration of the limb extremities than in the principal motor area, but the proximal limb muscles, whose basic function is or was locomotion, are well represented. Although not strictly true in anatomical terms, functionally the supplementary motor area can be regarded as controlling the red nucleus on its own side and hence the rubrospinal UMN, which crosses immediately after its origin. The cortex of the supplementary motor area is supplied by the anterior cerebral artery.

Experimental work in primates other than man has shown that after bilateral pyramidotomy, movements can still be elicited by stimulation of the principal motor area in the precentral gyrus, and that its somatotopic organization is unaffected. This is one of the reasons why it is difficult to disentangle some of the motor (but not the reflex) function of the corticobulbospinal and corticorubrospinal systems.

The *corticobulbospinal pathway* has three functions which may become disordered:

(a)   It brings about movements, particularly fine ('skilled') movements of the digits; such movements include reciprocal inhibition of antagonists.

(b)   It has an inhibitory action, as outlined above; during active normal voluntary movement, pyramidal inhibition suppresses movement not only of antagonist muscles, but also of neighbouring 'unwanted' muscles, so further refining and delimiting 'skilled' movement.

(c) It alone is responsible for the integrity of superficial reflexes evoked by low-intensity mechanical stimulation:

The four *abdominal reflexes*, whereby segments of the rectus abdominis contract when the skin overlying them is lightly stroked.

The *cremasteric reflex*, whereby the cremaster muscle contracts on stroking the skin on the inner aspect of the thigh. Although not often elicited in the course of a routine neurological examination, it may be useful (in the 50% of the human race in whom it may be tested) because the recti abdominis may be too flabby to give a reaction, even in a neurologically intact individual.

The *plantar reflex* consists of plantar flexion of the big toe on stroking the sole of the foot. This normal reflex may be regarded as part of a tactile placing reflex, whereby the lower limb moves down to obtain a stance on a supposed surface as soon as contact is registered on the outer border of the sole. It is not present in normal infants, but appears when walking is achieved.

Isolated lesions of the whole corticospinal tract are virtually unknown in man, though they have been surgically produced in patients with other types of upper motor neurone disease. In the chimpanzee, the most noticeable residual deficit following medullary pyramidotomy is replacement of fine finger movements (e.g. picking sweets out of a box) by awkward shovelling or scraping movements of the whole hand. It is therefore interesting that occasional cases of eighth nerve sheath tumour, in which it is possible that some compression of the medullary pyramid occurs, may complain of an inability to write.

The origin of the corticospinal system is damaged in lesions of the principal motor cortex. The most characteristic sign seen in this or any other lesion involving the pyramidal tract is replacement of the normal flexor plantar reflex by the *extensor plantar response* first described by Babinski, to whom this abnormal reflex is eponymously attributed. It consists of dorsiflexion of the big toe and fanning of the other toes on stimulation of the sole; and it is in fact the beginning of a withdrawal reflex. The extensor plantar response, when present, can often be elicited from a much wider area, including the front of the shin, than the normal flexor response. Experience with a large number of normal and abnormal cases shows that elicitation of the abnormal extensor response requires stimulation at higher intensity than does that of the normal flexor response. This is to be expected, for if the extensor response is the beginning of a withdrawal response, it will be activated by $A\delta$ (Group III) cutaneous afferents, whereas a tactile placing reaction such as the normal flexor plantar response will be activated from $A\beta$ (Group II) cutaneous afferents.

The extensor plantar response is such a sensitive indicator of damage to fibres issuing from the principal motor cortex that it may be seen, evanescently and bilaterally, in a very wide variety of cerebral insults; most unconscious patients, from whatever cause, have upgoing big toes. A further proviso must be added: the plantar response, normal or abnormal, is often very difficult or even impossible to elicit despite its cardinal importance in neurology. It is to be hoped that all readers of this work, if they cannot elicit a plantar response, will say so; and not, after looking at all the other signs and symptoms, write down that the patient has a big toe going in the direction in which it is felt that it ought to go!

The other superficial reflexes (abdominal and cremasteric) will simply be lost. If the pyramidal lesion is of sudden onset, as in cerebral artery thrombosis or a vascular accident in the internal capsule or spinal cord, the immediate result is flaccid hemiparesis (assuming the whole tract to be involved). In the case of cortical lesions confined to the principal motor area, the flaccid paresis, soon accompanied by the superficial reflex changes described, may be of long duration, or not even change to the hypertonic (spastic) type before recovery. However, in many cases involving the cortex, and all cases involving the corticospinal tract in the internal capsule, brainstem, and spinal cord, the paresis soon changes from the flaccid to the spastic type. This observation suggests that two functional types of corticospinal neurone, perhaps with different origins, may be concerned; and that in some cortical lesions only those fibres whose destruction causes flaccidity, and are responsible for the superficial reflexes, are involved; while at lower levels, due to anatomical propinquity, both types must inevitably be damaged together.

In cases of spastic paresis, a number of features can be recognized as due to the corticospinal lesion. Voluntary movements cannot be made or are made with great difficulty; the distal limb musculature, particularly in the hand, is most severely affected. Voluntary movements of the lower face are also impaired, but the forehead can usually be wrinkled because it is bilaterally represented in the cortex, and so can be controlled by upper motor neurones originating on the unaffected side. This is one of the ways in which it can be differentiated from a lower motor neurone lesion of the VIIth nerve (Chapter 1), for in the latter case the affected half of the brow is also paralysed. Another differentiating characteristic is that emotional movements of the face may be possible, and even exaggerated ('emotional lability') in pyramidal lesions, though they obviously cannot be performed when the final common pathway in the lower motor neurone is not working. The reason for the preservation of emotional movements is because they are under control of an upper motor neurone other than the corticobulbar fibres originating in the precentral gyrus; such movements may be exaggerated because of loss of the inhibitory control normally exerted by the interrupted UMN.

Disinhibition, as explained above, is an important characteristic of corticobulbospinal lesions. It is responsible for:

(a)   Reflex spasticity and exaggeration of the tendon jerks.

(b) The appearance of 'new' tendon jerks. The most characteristic of these is the jaw jerk, which is not usually present in normal individuals in whom tonic inhibitory control is intact.

(c) The appearance of more widespread reflex movements. This has already been referred to as exemplified by wrist flexion accompanying elicitation of the biceps jerk. A very interesting, because characteristic, example of this is *Hoffmann's sign*: when the terminal phalanx of the middle finger is flicked the forefinger and thumb oppose. When present, this sign is pathognomonic of a corticospinal lesion.

It is of course possible to encounter lesions which affect only part of the corticobulbospinal upper motor neurone. Such lesions are most likely, for anatomical reasons, to be in the cortex of the principal motor area, because of its wide extent, or in the spinal cord below the termination of many of the fibres; but sub-total lesions may also be less frequently encountered in the internal capsule and brainstem.

When a corticospinal lesion is of gradual onset, if it involves corticolumbar fibres, the patient may complain of heaviness and dragging of the leg; examination reveals that an extensor plantar response will have developed at an early stage. In spastic paresis of long standing, muscle wasting does not generally occur because the muscles are kept in trim by reflex activity, unlike in a lower motor neurone lesion. An exception must however be made for certain cases who have been bedridden for lengthy periods of time, in whom disuse atrophy may eventually appear. In recovery from spastic paresis, the residual (and often permanent) deficit of precision movements of the digits is a pathognomonic feature.

The *corticorubrospinal motor system* virtually never exhibits isolated lesions in its rubrospinal upper motor neurone. However, lesions of the supplementary motor area of the cortex, which controls the red nucleus, are encountered. As a workable simplification, it may be said that in the normal state, this whole system is chiefly responsible for locomotion; its influences are therefore chiefly but not entirely, exerted on proximal limb movements. When the system is dysfunctional, the resultant symptoms consist of a disinhibition—of the same physiological type as that seen in corticospinal lesions—of the lower motor neurones controlling proximal limb muscles, resulting in exaggeration of tendon reflexes and spasticity mainly affecting proximal limb muscles. The superficial reflexes dependent on the corticospinal system are not changed.

Consideration of cortical topography and arterial supply show that it would be almost impossible to have a lesion of the supplementary motor area without concomitant damage to the lower limb representation in the principal motor area; and this is in fact what happens in, for instance, anterior cerebral artery thrombosis or pressure from a falx meningioma. Such a lesion will cause supplementary motor corticorubrospinal symptoms in the upper limb, and combined corticorubrospinal plus corticospinal symptoms in the lower limb. Thus the lower limb will exhibit spasticity in both proximal and distal muscles, and an extensor plantar response, while in the upper limbs the spasticity is markedly greater in the proximal muscles, and there is no Hoffmann's sign. Another sign which when present is pathognomonic of a lesion of the supplementary motor area or of the part of area 6 lying on the lateral surface of the hemisphere in front of the principal motor area, is the grasp reflex, whereby the hand closes around an object drawn across the palm. The common experience of seeing a baby, before it can walk, standing upright in a play-pen and grasping the railings, allows us to interpret supplementary motor area lesions as knocking out locomotor function and uncovering the neural mechanisms which maintain a plastic upright posture.

It should be noted, that when the supplementary and

principal motor upper limb areas, or their efferents, are both put out of action, there is no grasp reflex; it becomes impossible because of the paresis (flaccid or spastic) of the hand. Hoffmann's sign may however be present in such cases of double motor system lesion.

The *vestibulospinal upper motor neurone arises from the lateral vestibular nucleus*, and is distinctive in two ways: it is uncrossed,\* and it acts almost exclusively on lower limb extensor (antigravity) lower motor neurones. It has already been explained that the latter action involves $\alpha$-motor neurones. Three influences on the lateral vestibular nucleus must be considered when attempting to explain clinical symptomatology (Fig. 1). These are excitation from the otolith organ (saccule and utricle of the vestibular apparatus), tonic inhibition indirectly from the cerebral cortex, and influences from the cerebellum (see Chapter 4).

When there is interference with input from the vestibular organ, as in Menière's disease, there may be sudden collapse of extensor tone, causing the sufferer to fall to the ground, to the side of the lesion. In sheath tumours of the vestibular nerve, there may be diminished tone on the ipsilateral side, causing deviation to the side of the lesion. Other symptoms of this condition are due to effects on eye movements through the medial longitudinal fasciculus, and are dealt with in Chapter 1.

The origin and course of corticovestibular influences is unknown. However, they must pass through the internal capsule, since this is the only way cortical efferents can get from the forebrain to lower centres (*vide infra*); and they must pass through the midbrain, where they are believed to relay in the interstitial nucleus of Cajal. Accidents (particu-

---

\* The reason for this is probably that the vestibular apparatus and its bulbospinal connections were evolved before the visual system; central pathways appearing in evolutionary time after the visual cross to compensate for optic decussation.

larly motor cycle accidents) may cause damage to the mid-brain by impaction against the edge of the tentorial notch; in cases which recover, it is believed that oedema subsequent to the contusion is responsible for compression of the tegmentum (causing loss of consciousness) and *decerebrate rigidity*. This is an extensor rigidity of the lower limbs, presumed to be due to functional discontinuity of tonic corticovestibular inhibition, and therefore to unopposed vestibulospinal facilitation of extensor LMNs. The position of the upper limbs in the midbrain syndrome is usually extended. Decerebrate rigidity should be distinguished from decorticate rigidity, in which the cortical origin of other motor systems is also damaged. In this condition, although the lower limbs also display extensor rigidity of vestibulospinal type, the upper limbs are usually flexed.

*Stroke* is probably the commonest single neurological syndrome which most medical practitioners encounter. It is generally caused by ischaemia in the internal capsule. Obviously the amount of neural tissue damaged or destroyed varies from case to case, but certain characteristic changes are common to every case. After an initial flaccid hemiplegia, thought to be due to shock, spastic hemiplegia develops. If the damage is sufficiently extensive, there is an upper motor neurone lesion of the face on the side opposite the lesion, together with loss of speech (Chapter 6), if the lesion is in the dominant hemisphere. The spastic hemiplegia of the body below the head is of course also on the side opposite the lesion. It is characterized by:
(a)  Loss of voluntary movements, spasticity, hyper-reflexia, and recruitment of reflex movements in the distal parts of the limb; loss of abdominal and cremasteric reflexes, extensor plantar response, and frequently appearance of Hoffmann's sign. All these are due to functional interruption of the corticospinal upper motor neurone.

(b)  Spasticity of proximal limb segments, due to functional interruption of corticorubral fibres.

(c)  Adoption of an extended position by the paretic lower limb, perhaps due to functional interruption of inhibitory cortico-interstitio-vestibular impulses.

It will be seen from the foregoing that three of the four central motor systems listed at the beginning of the chapter are involved. The reason why the fourth, the so-called extrapyramidal system, is not implicated is that many cortical influences on it are relayed through the basal ganglia, which are on either side of the internal capsule.

Just as stroke is the commonest symptom complex in neurology, so the commonest error in neurology is the belief that it is caused by a lesion of the pyramidal tract (i.e. efferents from the principal motor cortex) alone, and that it is unnecessary to invoke damage to other central motor systems. Corticobulbar and corticospinal fibres in fact occupy only a very small cross-sectional area in the genu and posterior limb of the internal capsule. Apart from the corticorubral and cortico-interstitio-vestibular fibres mentioned above, the internal capsule also contains descending corticopontine, corticotectal, corticoreticular, corticogracile, corticocuneate, and cortico-god-knows-what-else fibres. It also contains ascending thalamo-cortical fibres, and in fact there is quite frequently an element of sensory dysfunction in stroke; unless it is dramatic, it frequently passes unnoticed, and may be overlooked if not actively sought.

Bilateral degeneration, at cortical or capsular level, of pyramidal-type corticonuclear fibres brings about the condition of pseudobulbar palsy, which has some clinical features in common with the LMN disorder known as chronic bulbar palsy (Chapter 1). So far as the facial nerve is concerned, emotional movements are present and even exaggerated (disinhibited) in the UMN type of lesion (*vide supra*). While loss of supranuclear control of the last three cranial nerves leads to dysarthria and eventually to dysphonia the condition can clearly be differentiated from an LMN lesion by the absence of fibrillation in the tongue.

## THE BASAL GANGLIA AND ASSOCIATED NUCLEI
### (*IAPNS*, Fig. 48)

The upper motor neurones proper to the 'extrapyramidal system' are reticulospinal, but since the globus pallidus projects to the ventroanterior and ventrolateral thalamic nuclei (Fig. 3), the 'extrapyramidal system' also influences the output of the motor cortex through the corticospinal and corticorubrospinal systems. Like the vestibulospinal upper motor neurone, reticulospinal neurones are not recognizably involved alone in pathological states. However, syndromes caused by lesions in the basal ganglia and associated nuclei (notably the substantia nigra and the subthalamus) are relatively common. Extrapyramidal diseases (as it will be impossible to prevent this group of maladies being called), like other central motor system affections, cause changes in muscle tone, usually in the direction of hypertonia (rigidity); as explained above, reticulo-spinally mediated hypertonus is due to disinhibition of tonic $\gamma$-motor neurones, so is not accompanied by exaggeration of the tendon reflexes. They do not cause an inability to move (paresis), except in so far as rigidity may make movement difficult. What is really characteristic of these disease states is that *they are virtually always associated with spontaneous* (involuntary) *movements*, which are not seen in disorders of any other central motor systems. The spontaneous movements vary from tremor through the writhing movements of athetosis, the jerking of limbs (chorea) or head (spasmodic torticollis) to the violent movements of hemiballismus involving one whole side. This last is caused by a lesion, usually vascular, of the contralateral subthalamus, and may be fatally exhausting if not treated.

Because *Parkinson's disease* is by far the commonest 'extrapyramidal' disorder its pathophysiology may be used to illustrate the complexity of the system. The syndrome is due to degeneration of the dopaminergic nigro-striatal projection, and can be alleviated by replacement therapy. It is characterized by tremor at rest of the extremities and sometimes the head, at about 3 Hz; and reflex hypertonus of the whole musculature, including the face. Following the observation that Parkinsonian tremor, which mainly involves the hands and feet, disappeared on one side if sufferers underwent a subsequent stroke on the other side, elective surgical section proved that the tremor is in fact largely mediated by the corticospinal tract. It will be remembered that the globus pallidus, in addition to its downward projections, as simplistically illustrated in Fig. 3, also projects to ventral thalamic nuclear groups which influence the motor cortex. This provided the rationale for the operation of ventrolateral thalamotomy, which was extensively and reasonably successfully used for the relief of Parkinsonian symptoms before the discovery of the therapeutic effects of l-DOPA. The fact that ventrolateral thalamotomy has such a beneficial effect on Parkinsonian tremor, and indeed a number of other 'extrapyramidal' dyskinesias, implies that they are mediated by cortifugal systems, including the corticospinal, which are not themselves 'extrapyramidal'.

Given that most of the extrapyramidal disorders are due to degeneration in part of an interconnected nuclear system in forebrain, diencephalon, and midbrain, it would appear that dyskinesia results when an inbalanced output from these nuclei reaches the motor cortex. However, less is known about the physiology and pathophysiology of the 'extrapyramidal' system than of other central motor systems.

Within the *spinal cord*, the upper motor neurones of central motor systems may be destroyed by disease or injury. All descending (and ascending) systems may be interrupted by trauma and compression; while multiple sclerosis may eventually affect all upper motor neurones (as well as sensory pathways), although it tends in its terrible progression to involve more recently-evolved upper motor neurones (corticospinal, rubrospinal) before phylogenetically older ones (vestibulospinal, reticulospinal). System diseases such as amyotrophic lateral sclerosis, Friedreich's ataxy and subacute combined degeneration have a predilection for the lateral white columns containing the corticospinal and rubrospinal UMNs; though in the two latter, as already explained, concomitant involvement of the dorsal columns prevents the appearance of spasticity and hyper-reflexia.

Any of the conditions producing lateral column degeneration, if unrelieved, will progress to paraplegia-in-extension, in which the paraplegic lower limbs are extended due to still-intact vestibulospinal action. In the case of system disease such as multiple sclerosis in which all upper motor neurones are involved, or the later stages of spinal cord compression, which results in virtual transection, or traumatic transection itself,* paraplegia-in-flexion ensues by the time the vestibulospinal upper motor neurone is no longer functional, because in the absence of all descending control, only segmental flexion reflexes are left. Except in cases of sudden transection, therefore, paraplegia-in-extension precedes paraplegia-in-flexion.

The clinical significance of central motor systems may be summarized by considering *motor disintegration*. This process describes residual motor functions as the systems are successively stripped away in reverse order of evolutionary appearance:

(i) Removal of the pyramidal system abolishes long superficial reflexes (including placing reflexes) and skilled move-

---

* Acute transection of the spinal cord immediately results in spinal concussion (shock), in which the neural mechanisms of the spinal cord become completely functionless (so look out for acute retention of urine). After an interval, usually of weeks, autonomous cord functions reappear, together with paraplegia-in-flexion.

ments of the digits. It leaves a hyper-reflexic organism, capable of locomotion and postural adjustment.

(ii) Additional loss of corticorubrospinal function takes away the capacity for locomotion, and reduces the organism to an exaggerated ability for plastic stance, exemplified by increased tone, especially in proximal limb muscles, and a grasp reflex to help maintain the upright bipedal posture.

(iii) When only bulbospinal systems of reticular and vestibular origin remain intact, the organism maintains a rigid and invariable 'antigravity' (extensor) posture.

(iv) Finally only spinal flexor reflex activity is left; this stage is frequently heralded by the appearance of flexor spasms.

In addition to the upper motor neurones which have been discussed above, the spinal cord also contains descending bulbospinal fibres which control the activity of preganglionic autonomic neurones whose cell bodies lie in the inter-mediolateral 'columns' of the spinal grey matter. These descending fibres are of small diameter, and lie deep in the lateral columns of the spinal white matter (fig. 6). Both these factors mean that such fibres are relatively well-protected against extramedullary compression, so that they do not usually become affected until after severe signs of upper motor neurone disorders have developed. In intramedullary lesions, on the other hand, they may become involved at an early stage.

Lesions in the upper part of the spinal cord may affect descending control of the sympathetic outflow, resulting in changes in sweating and piloerection, which frequently go unnoticed, being of a relatively trivial nature. However, if the lesion is above the first thoracic segment, the more readily noticeable Horner's syndrome (constriction of the pupil, slight ptosis, enophthalmos, and anhidrosis of the face) may be present. But at any level down to and including the lumbar enlargement, disorder of sacral parasympathetic function may be caused, and this is far more important. The earliest symptom in the male is often impotence, but it is loss of bladder control, and later of rectal control, which are the gravest consequences. Once sphincter control has been lost, it is but rarely fully recovered. It is for this reason that it is essential for every medical practitioner to be aware of the earliest signs—'heavy' leg, paraesthesiae, foot drop—which may raise the suspicion of spinal cord compression. Early intervention, while it may fail to relieve such dysfunction as already has appeared, may well prevent the appearance of some of the most debilitating and degrading symptoms with which any patient can be afflicted.

Finally, it must be recalled that, for self-evident anatomical reasons, lesions in the lower brainstem or spinal cord, such as syringobulbia and syringomyelia, the myelopathy of cervical spondylosis, amyotrophic lateral sclerosis, intra-medullary tumours and vascular accidents, can bring about the simultaneous appearance of upper and lower motor neurone disorders. In such cases, if sensory signs are absent, the distribution of the uppermost LMN dysfunction will mark the level of the rostral border of the lesion, while UMN disorder will occur below this. In the spinal cord, upper and lower motor neurone lesions will be on the same side. But above the pyramidal decussation, the functional primacy of the corticospinal tract usually ensures that signs of UMN disorders occur on the side contralateral to the lesion, while the LMN signs are of course on the same side (see figs. 7-11).

# CHAPTER 3
## CENTRAL SOMATOSENSORY
## SYSTEMS AND SENSORY LEVELS

Subsequent to the penetration of the dorsal root into the spinal cord, ascending sensory fibres are segregated (separated) by size, synapsis, modality and laterality (*IAPNS*, Chapters 6 and 10). Large low-threshold mechanoreceptive primary afferents pass up the dorsal column without synapse; because they are uncrossed, the caudalmost fibres will be most medial and the rostralmost furthest lateral. The clinically-tested and testable-sensory modalities represented in the dorsal columns are: touch-pressure, joint position sense (kinaesthesia), and 'vibration sense' which is the para-esthesia experienced when large numbers of Pacini corpuscles are synchronously activated in phase with one another. Note that no non-mechanical modalities are represented in the dorsal columns.

The smaller primary afferent fibres in the dorsal root terminate in the grey matter of the dorsal horn in the segment of entry. After one or more synaptic relays, long axons cross the spinal cord obliquely and ascend in the contralateral anterolateral white columns. There are two components of the ascending anterolateral fibres: (a) spino-reticular (including palaeospinothalamic), subserving ill-defined 'protopathic' sensations which include erotic sensation, tickle, itch and 'real' pain (*IAPNS*, Chapter 11; and Chapter 7); and (b) the somatotopically-organized neospinothalamic tract, which mediates mechanoreceptive sensations of both middling

44

and high threshold—the latter being tested as pinprick sensation—and thermal sensation. Because the (neo) spinothalamic pathway is crossed, caudal segments are represented most laterally and rostral segments most medially. It should be noted that the number of spinothalamic fibres is small relative to the number of fibres in the dorsal columns, as well as to the number of spinoreticular fibres. As will be seen, the numerical disproportion between the two lemniscal pathways has some significance in clinical symptomatology. Note also that although temperature sensation and high threshold

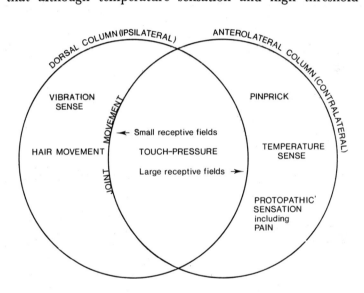

Fig. 5.  Clinical function of dorsal and anterolateral spinal columns. The left circle represents the functions of the dorsal column, the right those of the anterolateral column; the area of overlap in the mechano-sensitive range is shown. Joint movement, while principally represented in the dorsal column system, can sometimes be appreciated when only the anterolateral columns are intact. This function, as well as pinprick and temperature sensations are subserved by the neospino-thalamic component of the anterolateral column, while the much larger spinoreticular component is probably the substrate for a whole series of ill-defined sensations which include tickle, erotic sensation, itch, and real (tissue damage) pain.

mechanical sensation (pinprick) are represented in the neo-spinothalamic tract alone, what might be called middle-thres-hold mechanical sensations in the touch-pressure range, and perhaps some joint position sensation, are represented in both ipsilateral dorsal and crossed anterolateral columns (Fig. 5).

As a point of departure, the *Brown–Séquard syndrome* (Fig. 6) should be considered. It consists of a perfect hemi-section of the spinal cord, and, while the classical lesion can only be imagined as being executed upon a curarized victim by a berserk anatomist, elements of the Brown–Séquard syndrome are not infrequently met with in practice.

There are three essential factors to the full-fledged syndrome:

(a)   Loss of function in all upper motor neurones (Chapter 2) on the side of the lesion.

(b)   Loss of dorsal column sensory function on the side of the lesion and having its upper limit at the level of the lesion.

(c)   Loss of anterolateral column sensory function on the side opposite the lesion with its upper limit some four to six segments below the level of the lesion, due to the obliquity of the crossing. Sometimes the levels of thermanaesthesia and loss of pinprick sensation differ by a segment or so. but this is irregular in occurrence; similarly there is sometimes a band of hypoaesthesia* to noxious and thermal sensation above the level of complete loss. Both of these phenomena suggest that the degree of obliquity of individual crossing fibres frequently differs.

On the side of the lesion, there will be a retention of touch-pressure sensation, because some fibres mediating this sub-modality travel in the opposite (intact) spinothalamic tract (Fig. 5). Due to the fact that the spinothalamic pathway

---

* Bands of hyperaesthesia may also occur. They are described by some as being due to irritation. Beware. In this, and many (but not all) other instances where the word is used in neurological explanation, it appears to have little logical meaning. Many writers have, however, preferred to use it rather than admit that they do not understand the patho-physiological process in question.

contains fewer fibres than the dorsal column—medial lemniscus pathway, yet still has to carry representation of the whole body surface, it is obvious that the cortical receptive field for any given spinothalamic fibre will be larger than

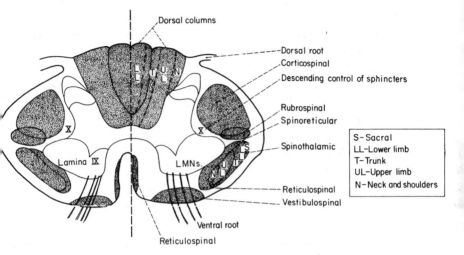

Fig. 6. The Brown–Séquard syndrome: destruction of one half of the spinal cord.

On the side of the lesion:
(a)   Lower motor neurone paralysis at the level of the lesion, together with a band of total sensory loss.
(b)   Upper motor neurone loss below the level of the lesion. Since all UMNs are involved in a complete lesion, there would be spastic monoplegia-in-flexion. On the other hand, sphincters would be unaffected, since descending controls are bilateral.
(c)   Loss of vibration sense, joint position sense, two-point discriminations from lesion of the dorsal columns (see Fig. 5).

On the side opposite the lesion:
(a)   Loss of pinprick, thermal, and true pain sensation, due to destruction of the neospino thalamic and spinoreticular pathways.

the cortical receptive field for a single fibre in the medial lemniscus. Since a cortical unit cannot distinguish more than one stimulus in its receptive field, the ability to discriminate two tactile stimuli depends upon excitation taking place in two (adjacent) fields. It follows that with the spinothalamic system functioning in the absence of the dorsal columns, two points will have to be further apart than normal for discrimination to be possible. This is often referred to as an 'impairment of two-point discrimination'. Every individual who intends to practise medicine should have two-point discrimination tested upon him/herself so that the wide variation between individuals can be appreciated, as well as the important intraindividual regional differences—between, for example, the finger pads and the back. This said, two-point discrimination should always be tested in symmetrical areas on the two sides of a patient's body; if there is a difference, a lesion of the dorsal columns, or medial lemniscus should be suspected on the side where the two points have to be further apart before they can be separately distinguished. Properly used, the two-point discrimination test is one of the most sensitive in neurology and a surer guide to dorsal column dysfunction than any other.

In the Brown–Séquard syndrome, in addition to the preservation of some mechanical sensitivity on the side of the lesion, it should be noted that there is no interference with cerebellar function, since while the dorsal spinocerebellar tract is ipsilateral, the ventral is crossed.

Incomplete Brown–Séquard syndromes are not uncommon, due not only to trauma but also to space-occupying lesions affecting the spinal cord. Since the penetrating sulcal branches of the anterior spinal artery supply either the left or the right half of the interior of the cord (*IAPNS*, Chapter 16), infarction of the area supplied by one such branch may be characterized by symptoms of the Brown–Séquard type; in such cases the dorsal columns are usually spared, since they are largely supplied from the posterior spinal arteries.

Because of the separation of fibres subserving different somatosensory sub-modalities within the spinal cord, it is obvious that incomplete lesions can lead to *dissociated sensory loss*. Because of their juxtaposition, bilateral lesions of the *dorsal columns* may be seen; and they may be afflicted by system diseases such as multiple sclerosis, subacute combined degeneration, Friedreich's ataxy, or tabes dorsalis. In such a case, the two-point discrimination test may be of little value since right-left differences may not be striking; very light tactile stimuli (as with a wisp of cotton wool) may be less certainly recognized than in an unaffected area. Loss of 'vibration sense' is a good indicator in the relatively young; but sensitivity to synchronous activation of Pacini corpuscles tends to disappear in the elderly. This leaves loss (usually partial) of joint position sense as the most reliable indicator; when bilaterally present and affecting input from the lower limbs, such loss is revealed by Romberg's test: the subject standing upright with eyes closed and heels and toes together can easily be disequilibrated by a sudden gentle push. This, however, has to be carefully differentiated from cerebellar disturbance, where spontaneous ataxy is usually present under such conditions.

While there is no doubt that conscious sensory changes occur in cases of dorsal column dysfunction under clinical conditions, there is at the present time considerable dispute about their basic physiological function; some argue that the principal role of the input from large low-threshold mechano-receptive fibres through the dorsal columns and medial lemniscus to the thalamus and principal somatic sensory cortex (SI) of the post-central gyrus is to provide feedback control for motor activity. This function of the low-threshold mechanoreceptive system is sometimes clinically evidenced by the presence of *imitation synkinesis* or *mirror movements*: in the presence of unilateral dysfunction of the afferent system, but with no motor deficit, a voluntary slow alternating movement (e.g. extension and flexion of wrist or ankle) on

the neurologically intact side is accompanied involuntarily
by similar movements on the side with the mechanoreceptive
deficit; but movements may be made on the deficient side
without anything happening on the sound side. This strange
symptom is not at all uncommon if looked for, and can occur
with an input lesion at any point from peripheral nerve to
post-central gyrus. It shows that this afferent system is
necessary to suppress bilaterally symmetrical movements
such as can normally be seen in infancy.

Lesions which affect one *anterolateral column*, such as
syringomyelia, will be marked by a contralateral inability to
distinguish the head from the point of a pin, thermanaesthesia,
and (usually but not always) loss of real pain sensation also.
Neighbouring upper motor neurones are frequently affected
at the same time.

It is from the distribution of sensory disturbance that it is
possible to estimate the localization, or at least the upper
limit, of a spinal cord lesion. The finding of a *sensory level*
will of course correlate with spinal cord segments, which in
the intact individual are invisible and impalpable. It is
therefore necessary to take the process a step further and
correlate the spinal cord and segments with the usually
palpable vertebral spines; or, in order to make sense of
radiographic, and particularly myelographic, evidence, with
vertebral bodies.

*Compression of the spinal cord* is most frequently due to
extramedullary pressure, and occasionally to an intramedullary process; some reference to this in relation to descending
fibres controlling sphincter function has been made in Chapter
2. To understand the compressive effects of an extramedullary
space-occupying lesion in the vertebral canal, it is necessary
to consider certain anatomical and physiological factors.
Firstly, since the spinal subarachnoid space is relatively
narrow, it will be obliterated between the tumour and the
spinal cord, so that there will be direct effects in the part of

the cord that is pressed against. Secondly, there will sometimes be a constriction effect at the level of the lesion. Since the cord as a whole has a certain elasticity, i.e. there is a small amount of extracellular space between the physiologically incompressible neural elements—the grey matter and deep white matter adjacent to it will be affected less than more superficially-placed fibres. Among the more superficial fibres, those of a larger diameter, i.e. the dorsal columns, are more likely to be affected than small axons, for the same reason as in peripheral nerve.

Of these two factors, the mechanical is the more important. It must be remembered, however, that, when the tumour is on the ventral aspect of the spinal cord, symptoms and signs of dysfunction in the dorsal part of the cord may be a leading feature because it and its supplying posterior spinal arteries are pressed against the posterior aspect of the vertebral canal. Furthermore, the anterior spinal artery is to some extent protected by its position within the ventral median sulcus, so that there is less tendency to ischaemia (which is the principal cause of myelopathy) in the ventral or anterior part of the spinal cord.

Lesions in the brainstem above the spinal cord produce a mixture of sensory and motor symptoms which may appear bizarre, but which in fact depend on a combination of the relationship of pathways, nuclei and the distribution of arteries—for such lesions are frequently vascular. While the key to the anatomical localization of such lesions is to identify the ipsilateral lower motor neurone or sensory nuclear disorder, it is probably conceptually simpler to consider the symptoms which would arise from hemisection of the brainstem at various levels (Figs. 7, 8, 9 and 10), and thus by eliminating those dysfunctions which are not present, to determine the true extent of the lesion. Even when a particular pathway or system is involved, the distribution of the appropriate changes below the level may be subtotal because of the patchy nature of vascular lesions.

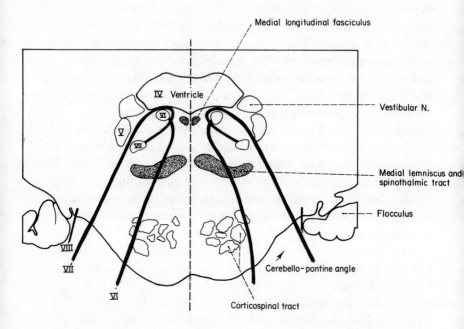

Medial longitudinal fasciculus

IV Ventricle

Vestibular N.

Medial lemniscus and spinothalmic tract

Flocculus

Cerebello-pontine angle

Corticospinal tract

Fig. 7.  Hemisection of the brainstem at the ponto-medullary junction would lead to:

On the side of the lesion
(a)  Lower motor neurone paralysis of the muscles of facial expression, through destruction of the intracerebral seventh nerve and its nucleus.
(b)  Paralysis of ocular abduction, due to loss of function in the sixth nerve nucleus.
(c)  Thermanaesthesia and analgesia of the face because the descending tract of the trigeminal nerve is destroyed.
(d)  Some hypertonus, particularly in proximal limb muscles, due to rubrospinal upper motor neurone damage.

On the side opposite the lesion
(a)  Paresis of gaze towards the affected side (i.e. medially) because of damage to the medial longitudinal fasciculus.
(b)  Loss of all somatic sensation in the body and limbs, due to destruction of the spinothalamic tract and superjacent tegmentum and the medial lemniscus. Since the latter is further medial, it is more likely to be spared than the pathways responsible for pain and temperature sensation.
(c)  Corticospinal upper motor neurone symptoms.

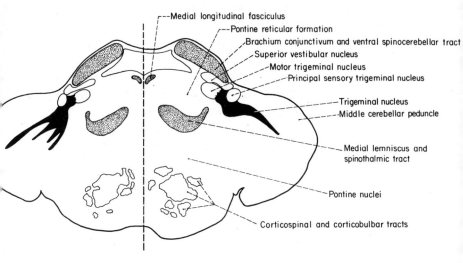

Fig. 8. Hemisection of the pons at the level of the motor trigeminal nucleus would lead to:

On the side of the lesion
(a)  Lower motor neurone paralysis of the muscles of mastication, due to the lesion of the motor trigeminal nucleus.
(b)  Proximal limb muscle hypertonus from interference with the rubrospinal upper motor neurone.
(c)  Paralysis of gaze towards the side of the lesion because of damage to the medial longitudinal bundle.
(d)  Loss of mechanoreceptive sensation in the face due to destruction of the principal sensory nucleus of the trigeminal nerve.
(e)  Cerebellar symptoms, including tremor (see Chapter 4) because of damage to the brachium conjunctivum.

On the side opposite the lesion
(a)  Corticospinal upper motor neurone symptoms including the the muscles of facial expression, palate and tongue.
(b)  Hemianalgesia and therm-anaesthesia of the face because the crossed ascending projection from the descending trigeminal nucleus is damaged.
(c)  Loss of all somatic sensation in the body due to involvement of medial lemniscus, spino-thalamic tract and ascending reticular pathways.

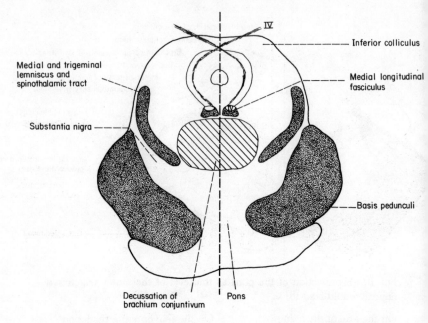

FIG. 9. Hemisection of the midbrain at the level of the inferior colliculus (NB. this is at, or above, the level of the tentorial notch) would lead to:

On the side of the lesion
(a) Lower motor neurone paralysis of the superior oblique muscle of the eye, because of damage to the trochlear nerve nucleus.

On the side opposite the lesion
(a) Upper motor neurone paresis of both pyramidal and rubrospinal type, including the face and head.
(b) Loss of all somatic sensation including the face.

(i) Bilateral paralysis of conjugate downward gaze due to destruction of the medial longitudinal fasciculus.
(ii) Cerebellar symptoms, including tremor (see Chapter 4) on one or both sides because of damage to the decussating brachium conjunctivum.

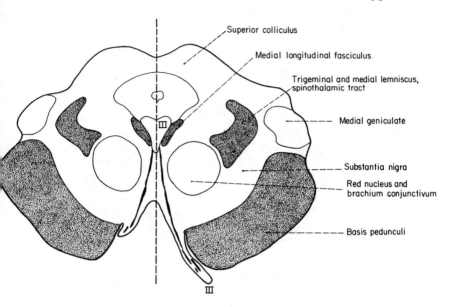

FIG. 10. Hemisection of the midbrain at the level of the superior colliculus (NB. this is supratentorial) would lead to:

On the side of the lesion
(a)   Third nerve paralysis, including pupillary dilation, of lower motor neurone type.

NB  Parkinsonian-type symptomatology may occur if the pars compacta of the substantia nigra is involved, and/or hemiballismus if the subthalamic nucleus (corpus Luysii) is damaged; but both these would be virtually symptomless if UMN signs are present.

On the side opposite the lesion
(a)   Paresis of upward gaze due to lesion of medial longitudinal fasciculus.

(b)   Upper motor neurone signs of combined pyramidal and rubrospinal type, affecting face as well as body.

(c)   Cerebellar-type symptoms from destruction of the crossed brachium conjunctivum; these would not be evident with concomitant UMN damage.

(d)   Loss of all somatic sensory modalities over face and body due to interruption of medial lemniscus, spinothalamic tract, and ascending reticular pathways.

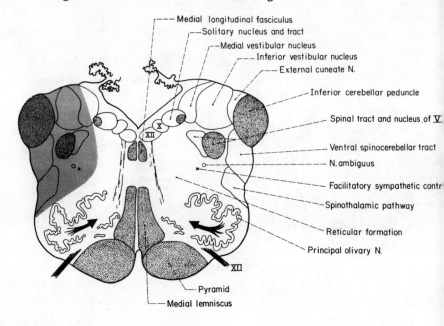

FIG. 11. Lateral medullary syndrome due to necrosis in the shaded area; there would be:

On the side of the lesion
(a) analgesia and therm-anaesthesia of the face due to destruction of the descending tract and nucleus of V.
(b) Lower motor neurone paralysis of the palate and larynx, leading to dysphagia and dysarthria, from affection of the nucleus ambiguus.
(c) Horner's syndrome, particularly pupillary constriction, from loss of descending control on the upper thoracic sympathetic outflow.
(d) Nystagmus due to affection of the vestibular nuclei.

On the side opposite the lesion
(a) Analgesia and therm-anaesthesia of the trunk and limbs due to interruption of ascending spinothalamic and spinoreticular fibres; this is occasionally accompanied by spontaneous ('thalamic') pain in the analgesic half of the body (see Chapter 7).

An exception to the rule of considering theoretical hemi-section must be made for the medulla oblongata, because extensive lesions in this region are fatal due to involvement of bulbospinal and lower motor neurones controlling vital functions. At this level, therefore, it is more profitable to consider the lateral medullary (Wallenberg's) syndrome, which is caused by ischaemia in the territory of the posterior inferior cerebellar artery (Fig. 11); greater or lesser extents of damage are described in relation to the figure.

---

(e)   Cerebellar-type symptoms (see Chapter 4) due to involvement of the inferior cerebellar peduncle (restiform body).

If the lesion extends further ventrally and medially than shown, there would also be:

(f)   Lower motor neurone paralysis of the tongue from damage to the hypoglossal nerve.

(b)   Cerebellar-type symptoms (see Chapter 4) because of inferior olivary involvement, perhaps hidden by:

(c)   Corticospinal upper motor neurone symptoms from affection of the medullary pyramid above its decussation.

# CHAPTER 4
# THE CEREBELLUM AND
# POSTERIOR FOSSA

The cerebellum may be divided rostro-caudally into anterior, posterior and flocculo-nodular lobes, and medio-laterally into vermis, intermediate, and lateral zones (*IAPNS*, Chapter 14). In the clinical context, it is the mediolateral functional organization which is most important. It will be recalled that the three zones of cerebellar cortex project respectively onto the fastigial, globose and emboliform (interposed), and dentate nuclei; and that these nuclei in their turn influence upper motor neurones, either by facilitating them or by not facilitating them (but never by inhibiting them). Afferents to the cerebellum are of three types: descending via the pontine nuclei from the motor cortex (representing the pyramidal system) and via the inferior olivary nucleus from the red nucleus and basal ganglia (representing the 'extrapyramidal system'); ascending, via the spinocerebellar tracts which convey information about the state of muscle tension (proprioception) to the cerebellar cortex, in such wise that axial (trunk) musculature is represented on the vermis and the extremities laterally; thirdly, there are two way connections between the vestibular nuclei (influenced by information about axial equilibrium from the vestibular apparatus) and the cerebellar vermis, fastigial nucleus, and flocculus.

Functionally, the cerebellum is a servocontrol mechanism superimposed on upper motor neurones. It is concerned with muscle tone, so with posture; and with muscular co-ordination, so with movement. In essence, the cerebellum compares information it receives from descending afferents about intent to contract muscles with information about the actual state of contraction from musculotendinous afferents and about actual position from vestibular afferents; performs a computation on the basis of two types of data, and through its output influences upper motor neurones with respect to the next component of muscular adjustment. Inputs to the cerebellum, and its output to the vestibular nuclei are uncrossed. Outputs to other upper motor neurones are crossed, but since these UMNs themselves decussate as they descend, the net result in the final analysis is that *all cerebellar effects are ipsilateral.*

Disorders of the cerebellum may be extrinsic, such as tumours on the sheaths of the fifth or eight nerves in the cerebello-pontine angle (Fig. 7) which may compress the cerebellum from its inferolateral aspect, or tumours in the fourth ventricle which abut on its under surface. Intrinsic disorders may be degenerative, or consist of a new growth, abscess, or vascular anomaly. Lesions of the cerebellum are always associated with a reduction in the resting tone of muscles. This is because the normal intact cerebellum may facilitate upper motor neurones, but never inhibits them,* so that hypertonus cannot result from the removal of cerebellar influences on UMNs. The decreased tone of cerebellar disease is seen as floppiness on shaking relaxed joints, increased pendular movement of the arm(s) on tapping the outstretched hand, or falling away of a limb extended against gravity (both the latter tests should be applied with the eyes closed). Unlike minor degrees of motor neurone disorder, hypotonus of

* In fact, some inhibitory Purkinje cells of the cortex in the anterior lobe vermis do pass directly to the lateral vestibular nucleus so the statement is not absolutely true. But this effect is not seen in clinical practice. Experimentally, decerebrate rigidity of vestibular nuclear origin is made worse by destruction of the anterior lobe vermis.

cerebellar origin is not felt by the subject as 'weakness'—
which may help to serve as a reminder that the cerebellum
is not a motor centre, but a servocontrol.

Loss of this control is expressed differently according to
whether the lateral region or the vermal zone are affected.
In the case of lateral cerebellar lesions involving the dentate
nucleus, or its efferents in the brachium conjunctivum, the
most striking and pathognomonic feature is 'intention tremor'
of the extremities (only one limb may be affected). This is a
scanning tremor only seen on movement, for the cerebellum
feeds on movement. It may be noted particularly at the end

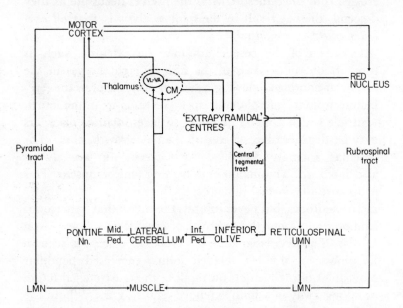

FIG. 12. Lateral cerebellar syndrome. The main connections of the
lateral cerebellum are shown. It can be seen that the chief inputs are from
the corticospinal and corticorubrospinal systems via the pontine and
olivary nuclei respectively, while its main output is from the dentate
nucleus to the cortical origin of these systems, via the ventrolateral and
ventroanterior thalamic nuclei (VL–VA) and the nucleus centrum
medianum thalami (CM). Lateral cerebellar symptomatology is thus
particularly seen as dyskinesia involving the limbs.

of a movement, such as the finger–nose or heel–shin tests, where it is described as dysmetria or past-pointing. Cerebellar tremor is in almost total contrast to the tremor at rest of basal ganglion ('extrapyramidal') disease. The circuits involved in the lateral cerebellar syndrome are illustrated in Fig. 12.

When the cerebellar vermis is involved (Fig. 13), loss of control is expressed as difficulty with balance, or ataxia. The gait is typically broad-based, and there is a tendency to lurch—when the disease process also involves one lateral lobe as well as the vermis then the lurching and tendency to

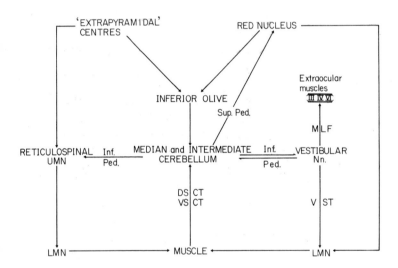

FIG. 13. Medial cerebellar syndrome. The main inputs to the medial cerebellum are the vestibular nuclei, the basal ganglia and red nucleus via the inferior olive, and peripheral stretch receptors via the dorsal (DSCT) and ventral (VSCT) spinocerebellar tracts. Outputs are to reticulospinal, rubrospinal, and vestibulospinal (VST) UMNs, and to vestibulo-ocular control mechanisms via the medial longitudinal fasciculus (MLF). Thus dysfunction of the median cerebellum will be chiefly expressed as changes of tone in postural muscle (hypotonia), and inco-ordination of locomotory (ataxia) and extraocular ('cerebellar nystagmus') muscles.

overbalance are towards the affected side. Tremor is seen in two axial structures—the voice-producing mechanism and the eyes. Cerebellar dysarthria is typically a drunken-sounding slurring of the voice, due to loss of feedback control of the vocalizing muscles. Dysmetria of the muscles controlling eye movements is expressed as a form of nystagmus; it depends on interruption of the connections between the vermal cortex and fastigial nuclei with the vestibular nuclei, and will be more fully discussed below.

The symptoms of midline cerebellar disorders, including nystagmus, are similar to those of acute alcoholic poisoning, a state with which students of medicine are traditionally supposed not to be entirely unfamiliar. This is no coincidence, for it is indeed the cerebellum which is the most susceptible part of the brain to alcohol, although the cerebral cortex is also affected. The cerebellum is also particularly sus-ceptible, sometimes in irreversible fashion, to some other forms of chemical insult.

## THE CEREBELLUM AND EYE MOVEMENTS

The vestibulospinal upper motor neurone, arising from the lateral vestibular nucleus, has been dealt with in Chapter 2. The semicircular canals, sensitive to angular acceleration in each of the three planes of space, project principally onto the superior vestibular nucleus, which reaches up into the inferior cerebellar peduncle as the latter turns up at right angles into the cerebellum. The medial longitudinal fasciculus (Figs. 1 and 2), connecting the vestibular complex with the VIth, IVth and IIIrd nerve nuclei (among others) receives projections from both the cortex of the flocculo-nodular lobe and the fastigial nuclei. Thus it may correctly be expected that eye movements will be affected when the axial cere-bellum (posterior lobe vermis, nodulus, and fastigial nucleus) or the flocculus are involved in disease process.

The flocculus is compressed by cerebello-pontine angle

tumours; since most of these arise from the sheath of the vestibular nerve, and/or also compress the vestibular nuclei, it is impossible, in practical terms, to disentangle a theoretical 'floccular syndrome' from symptoms due to involvement of the vestibular nerve and nuclei (see Chapter 1).

Median or paramedian cerebellar lesions, on the other hand, may not, at least in the first instance, involve extra-cerebellar structures. Such lesions cause an ocular intention tremor, which is more marked on looking to the side of the lesion. Cerebellar 'nystagmus' which is usually a lateral conjugate movement of the eyes does not occur at rest, but only on directing the gaze; in other words, it is an intention tremor. This ocular tremor is often called, probably wrongly, 'cerebellar nystagmus'. As mentioned in Chapter 1, it may be accompanied by a form of vertigo in which both the subject and external objects appear to be rotating away from the side of the lesion.

## EFFECTS ON CEREBELLUM OF INPUT LESIONS

While the dorsal spinocerebellar tract is ipsilateral through-out, the ventral tract decussates in the spinal cord, and again in the cerebellum (*IAPNS*, Chapters 6 and 14). The practical result of this is that a unilateral cord lesion, such as the Brown–Séquard syndrome, produces no symptoms of cerebellar type. However, a lesion which affects both spino-cerebellar tracts bilaterally such as some cases of Friedreich's ataxy, will be characterized by intention tremor of minor degree.

Unilateral lesions of the inferior cerebellar peduncle, which contains both a dorsal spinocerebellar tract and olivo-cerebellar fibres, will also cause cerebellar-type symptoms on the side of the lesion. Experimental lesions of the inferior olive give rise principally to ataxy and hypotonia, which is in good accord with the locomotory function of the rubrospinal UMN and the postural function of the 'extrapyramidal' system which both project to the cerebellum via the inferior olive.

Experimental lesions of the middle cerebellar peduncle, containing only ponto-cerebellar fibres, bring about disorders of movement, which are particularly marked in the extremities. This is equally in keeping with the association between the pyramidal UMN and the pontine nuclei. Cerebellar-type symptoms, affecting the contralateral extremities, are sometimes seen in man when the frontal cortical areas which project to the pontine nuclei are damaged.

## THE POSTERIOR FOSSA

Space-occupying lesions in the posterior cranial fossa are frequently due to pathology in the cerebellum. Another common cause is nerve sheath tumour, which nearly always occurs on the eighth nerve. While either of these will in the first instance cause symptoms proper to itself, further symptoms arise from compression of the lower brainstem, which prove fatal unless the cause is relieved.

Some of the symptoms of brainstem compression are also seen in cases of supratentorial space-occupying lesion (see Chapter 5), but they develop much more rapidly when the posterior fossa is the seat of the trouble. *Headache* is believed to be due to stretching of the richly-innervated meninges. *Drowsiness*, which later proceeds to unconsciousness, is thought to be due to affection of the ascending reticular activating system in the tegmental core of the brainstem. It should be noted that 'drowsiness' is a term employed by patients or their relatives, and adopted by members of the medical and nursing professions. What in fact happens is that affection (at first reversible) of the ascending reticular system brings about a decreased level of consciousness or *arousability*, so that the subject, unlike the normal dozer, cannot be snapped into alert wakefulness by the usual domestic stimuli.

*Vomiting*, an early feature of posterior fossa compression, is explained as being due to irritation of the vagal nuclei in the floor of the fourth ventricle. The medulla oblongata contains so-called 'centres' controlling vital functions such as respiration and cardiac activity. These are in fact reticulospinal neurones originating in the regions of the vagal and solitary nuclei, for central control systems know nothing of the anatomist's distinction between 'somatic' and 'autonomic' peripheral systems. It is loss of function in these descending pathways which is eventually fatal. An earlier sign, however, is due to loss of function in the bulbospinal neurones controlling the sympathetic outflow from the intermediolateral column of the spinal grey matter. This is *constriction of the pupil*, due to the unopposed action of the parasympathetic constrictor fibres in oculomotor nerve. The importance of this is that *pupillary constriction of central origin is always due to an intrabulbar* (posterior fossa) *lesion*. It must of course be borne in mind that a peripheral sympathetic lesion can also give rise to pupillary constriction; but it is unlikely that such a peripheral lesion will be accompanied by signs of an intracranial space-occupying lesion. Furthermore, the constricted pupil of peripheral origin is usually unilateral, that of brainstem origin bilateral.

# CHAPTER 5
# RAISED INTRACRANIAL PRESSURE AND HYDROCEPHALUS

The cranium is to all intents and purposes a closed box, containing (a) nervous tissue, (b) cerebrospinal fluid, and (c) blood. The nervous tissue is, under physiological conditions, of unvarying volume. Under pathological conditions, it may diminish in volume through atrophy, or increase by swelling or through the presence of a new growth. For practical purposes, cerebrospinal fluid (*IAPNS*, Chapter 3) may be regarded as being formed in the ventricles and removed from the subarachnoid space. In cases of cerebral atrophy its quantity increases to fill the space left by the diminishing forebrain. In the case of an increase in the volume of the brain or other non-cerebral intracranial contents, an adjustment in the quantity of cerebrospinal fluid can be made over time by increased absorption or diminished production. But since the total quantity of the fluid is normally only 120–150 ml, and since it cannot be entirely got rid of (particularly from the ventricles), change in its volume can only make a difference of considerably less than 10 % in the total intracranial volume of about 1500 ml.

The third constituent, blood, however, passes freely in and out of the cranial cavity. An increase in (a) or (b) or the presence of extravascular intracranial blood (*vide infra*) will inevitably result in a reduction of the quantity of blood flowing into and out of the brain. A delicate balance exists between the rapidly adjustable blood flow and the more slowly adjustable cerebrospinal fluid volume. This balance provides a certain degree of dynamic compensation for an increase in intracranial volume. But it has a limit which may be reached quite suddenly. This is why an intracranial lesion which has been slowly increasing in size over a considerable time may declare itself with dramatic suddenness instead of by slowly progressive symptoms from the start.

When the compensating mechanism breaks down, an increase in intracranial pressure occurs. While this brings about the symptoms to be described below, the ultimate result is due to cerebral anoxia from decreased blood flow; and this is the cause of death in the end. The usual cause of an increase in intracranial pressure is the presence of space-occupying lesion (SOL) which may be a new growth, an abscess, a parasitic cyst, or non-circulating blood. The last-named should be considered in terms of the anatomical origin and position of the blood vessels in the head.

The *middle meningeal artery* belongs to the external carotid circulation and therefore *cannot be directly visualized by internal carotid or vertebral angiography*. It lies in a groove (sometimes a canal) in the bone of the inner table of the diploë, outside the dura mater. When traumatically ruptured, usually by a skull fracture, the bleeding peels the dura away from the inside of the cranium. This *extradural haemorrhage* usually develops very rapidly, compressing and acutely displacing the brain deep to the deformable but inelastic dura, leading to early loss of consciousness.

The superior cerebral veins which drain into the superior sagittal sinus pierce the arachnoid before entering the intradural sinus. It is in this position that they may be torn by shearing forces consequent upon even a relatively mild head injury, often unaccompanied by skull fracture. Venous bleeding at this point occurs between the deep surface of the dura mater and the arachnoid, dissecting the arachnoid from the dura and forming a *subdural haematoma*. The venous haemorrhage may be an oozing rather than a frank bleed, so that a subdural haematoma may form and produce its compressive effects, insidiously and over a long time; it is frequently only to be differentiated from a new growth by its curiously fluctuant course.

The circle of Willis and its main branches are in the subarachnoid space. Aneurysms (which even in the un-ruptured state may act as SOLs*) on these vessels may bleed into the subarachnoid space. *Subarachnoid haemorrhage* may also occur over the cortical surface due to bleeding from a so-called arterio-venous malformation, which is actually a localized persistence of the cerebral arterio-venous fistulae of the early embryo. Due to spreading irritation of the well-innervated leptomeninges,† the onset of bleeding into the subarachnoid space is marked by a headache of a type which the subject has never before experienced, followed by general, and in some cases later by local, signs of compression.

Lastly, *intracerebral haemorrhage*—the presence of blood within the substance of the brain—may occur when bleeding from a ruptured aneurysm bursts into the cerebrum, or as the result of the rupture of an intracerebral vessel. In either case, the destruction of brain tissue is more important than pressure effects.

The brain and cerebrospinal fluid constitute, in physical terms, a single phase, so that the pressure of one is the pressure of the other. Cerebrospinal fluid can be tapped either in the lumbar theca, below the spinal cord—where, particularly in cases of arthritic spine, difficulty may be experienced in

* SOL—Space-occupying lesion; any abnormality taking up space in the craniovertebral system—not necessarily (but including) a neoplasm.

† Reflex stiffness of the posterior neck muscles occurs when the under-lying leptomeninges of the cisterna magna are irritated, and may be seen in both subarachnoid haemorrhage and (infective) meningitis. Sick people adopt the recumbent posture, which causes the appropriate irritants to pool in the cisterna magna.

inserting a needle between the vertebral laminae—or, more easily, in the cisterna magna through the atlanto-occipital membrane. In this latter site, care must be taken not to penetrate the medulla oblongata, but this can be avoided by using a needle with a guard on it. When cerebrospinal fluid is allowed to flow into an open vertical tube through the needle, what is measured is in fact the quantity of fluid displaced, and though related to pressure, its height in the 'manometer' varies with the diameter of the latter, since the total normal volume of cerebrospinal fluid is relatively small (120 ml); variations also occur due to the position of the patient. True pressure can be measured by attaching the needle to a strain gauge or a capacitance manometer. Normal fluid pressure or displacement is rapidly and greatly raised by jugular compression (Queckenstedt's test). If this manoeuvre produces no effect through a lumbar needle, it is evidence of a block within the spinal subarachnoid space. The immediate rise in quantity of fluid displaced on jugular compression is due to the increase in intracranial volume caused by the swelling (i.e. change from ellipsoid to circular cross-sectional area) of the cerebral veins. Any later rise is caused by diminution in the rate of cerebrospinal fluid absorption through the engorged veins, if the jugular pressure is maintained (which it should not be).

The symptoms of a rapid generalized rise in intracranial pressure are (a) headache—presumably due to tension on (stretching of) the richly-innervated dura mater; (b) drowsiness, and (c) nausea and vomiting—both probably caused by compression of the brainstem (Chapter 4 and below), (d) slowing of the heart rate* (bradycardia), reflexly set up by back pressure on the pressure receptors in the carotid sinus due to the increased resistance to arterial inflow into the

* Except in cases of sudden and rapid increases of intracranial pressure (e.g. in intracranial haemorrhage) this sign is very inconstant. When pressure increases more slowly, compensatory mechanisms such as a decrease in cerebral blood flow come into play.

cranial cavity; and (e) papilloedema. The most important
single sign is papilloedema (Chapter 1). This occurs because
of course the optic nerve and retina are part of the brain,
contained in the same meningeal sac; therefore the pressure
in and surrounding the optic nerve is the same as the pressure
in the brain, and oedema of one is reflected in oedema of the
other. Other signs may occur because of stretching of two
of the long cranial nerves (IV, VI) which supply the extra-
ocular muscles. Since lesions of the trochlear nerve cannot
easily be detected, lateral rectus palsy as a result of an
abducent nerve lesion is usually the first disorder to be seen.

Anatomically three cranial fossae are described, but the
tentorium cerebelli effectively divides the cranial cavity into
an infratentorial posterior fossa and a supratentorial region
comprising the middle and anterior fossae of topographical
anatomy. The volume of the posterior fossa, containing the
lower brainstem and cerebellum is very much smaller than
that of the supratentorial middle and anterior fossae,
containing the upper brainstem and cerebral hemispheres.
Thus an SOL of given size occupies a proportionately greater
volume, and produces proportionately greater effects, in the
infratentorial than in the supratentorial region; it is also
likely, at a relatively early stage, to obstruct cerebrospinal
fluid outflow. The practical results are that a posterior fossa
SOL (see Chapter 4) may cause general pressure effects
including papilloedema, before any localizing signs are seen;
whereas supratentorial SOLs frequently produce local
effects (see Chapter 6) before there is any evidence of
generalized pressure increase. There is, however, a special
cause of brainstem compression in the case of a supratentorial
SOL: this is *tentorial* (incisural) *herniation*. The cortical uncus,
which normally lies just above the tentorial notch, may be
forced down through it, as can be clearly seen by the
markings in fatal cases. Tentorial herniation has as its
principal clinical effect compression of the central reticular
core of the upper brainstem resulting in lowering of the level

of arousal (i.e. consciousness). Mention should also be made of hemiparesis which can occur as a result of compression of the cerebral peduncle (see Chapter 6).

## HYDROCEPHALUS

'Water on the brain' is strictly defined as an increase in the volume of the cerebrospinal fluid. Given the well-known abhorrence of nature for a vacuum, a decrease in the volume of the brain, such as occurs in atrophy, is compensated by an increase in the quantity of cerebrospinal fluid, without any increase in its pressure. Normal-pressure hydrocephalus in cases of this sort is merely the passive accompaniment of cerebral atrophy, which is itself frequently associated with arteriopathic dementia. Hydrocephalus is regarded as a pathological process in its own right when, in addition to volume increase, cerebrospinal fluid pressure is intermittently or chronically increased. Intermittent increase in pressure may be clinically indistinguishable from normal-pressure hydrocephalus unless continuous pressure recording is undertaken; as the treatment and prognosis of the two conditions are entirely different, it is of practical importance to be able to distinguish between them.

Since under normal conditions, the net rate of formation must equal the net rate of removal, an increase in volume and therefore of pressure must be due to either an increase in the rate of formation or a decrease in the rate of removal. As a cause of hydrocephalus, the first in its pure form is extremely rare, and occurs only when there is an active secretory *papilloma of the choroid plexus*. However, relative over-production can occur when there is an obstruction to free communication between the ventricles and the subarachnoid space, because the choroid plexus-containing ventricles produce more fluid than they absorb, while the converse is true of the subarachnoid space. *Obstructive hydrocephalus*, usually associated with *stenosis of the cerebral aqueduct* in the midbrain is by far the commonest form of the condition, and is essentially a disorder of infancy (obstructive hydrocephalus = infantile hydrocephalus). An anatomically similar condition is occasionally seen in adults when the (rostral) entrance to the aqueduct is blocked by a tumour of the third ventricle, acting as a ball-valve of the type encountered in a familiar item of domestic equipment. It should be noted that in both these forms of obstructive hydrocephalus, the fluid-containing space is divided into two compartments: an upper consisting of the first three ventricles and a lower comprising the fourth ventricle and craniospinal subarachnoid space. Theoretically (and very rarely in practice), obstructive hydrocephalus could arise from blockage of the outflow from the fourth ventricle, through the foramina of Luschka and Magendie.

In contrast to obstructive hydrocephalus, *communicating hydrocephalus*, the commonest form in adults, occurs when, although there is no obstruction to the free flow of cerebrospinal fluid, the transmeningeal absorptive mechanism fails to function properly, due for example to chronic arachnoiditis which may be caused by antecedent subarachnoid haemorrhage, often of minor degree, or by earlier acute meningitis; but is sometimes of unknown origin.

Because pressure changes are transmitted equally throughout the closed craniovertebral space, the symptoms and signs of hydrocephalus are essentially similar whichever of the above anatomical defects is the cause, being those of raised intracranial pressure. Differential diagnosis depends on a consideration of the patient's age plus special procedures such as ventriculography and/or pneumoencephalography, or computerized tomography. However, again due to anatomical differences, there are important differences between infantile and adult forms. In the infant in whom fusion of the cranial sutures has not yet occurred, the first sign (frequently undetected) of raised intracranial pressure is tension over, and bulging of, the anterior fontanelle; this is followed by an abnormal rate of increase in skull circumference.

Obviously, subsequent to closure of the fontanelles and fusion of the sutures (say after the age of 2 years), these changes are not seen.

Although most cases of hydrocephalus are treated by a shunt operation (ventriculo-cisternal, ventriculo-atrial, theco-peritoneal), not all are dealt with at an early stage, and it is important to understand the pathophysiology of the untreated condition in order to comprehend the changes which occur in the later stages of the disease, as well as those taking place in cases of space-occupying cerebral lesions.

A rise in cerebrospinal fluid pressure must be accompanied by a rise in cerebral venous pressure, in order that the unsupported leptomeningeal and cerebral veins may remain patent, leading eventually to a rise in pressure of the intra-dural venous sinuses into which they drain. The rise in venous pressure leads to interference with cerebral blood flow rates, and thus to (partial) anoxia. Owing to its less rich blood supply, white matter is affected by this before grey. In fact the ventricles enlarge at the expense of the white matter of the cerebral hemispheres, leading to a (sometimes very great) reduction of the distance between the ventricular wall and the external surface of the hemi-sphere. This is known as 'cortical thinning' although in reality the cerebral cortex itself, thanks to its rich blood supply, is unaffected until the final stages, and the intelli-gence of grossly hydrocephalic children may be quite normal. Death eventually supervenes when venous pressure is no longer able to overcome cerebrospinal fluid pressure, and so cerebral blood flow and hence tissue oxygenation fall to levels below those compatible with life.

However, it is evident that the rise in cerebrospinal fluid pressure opposes the secretion pressure of the choroid plexuses. This may be seen by the fact that the net rate of fluid formation falls as the pressure rises. Thus a state of equilibrium may be reached when formation is sufficiently reduced by back-pressure to equal removal. Such cases are said to undergo spontaneous arrest. Such arrest is prima facie more likely to occur in communicating hydrocephalus, but is certainly not unknown in obstructive hydrocephalus.

*Practical note.* When the source of increased pressure is in the cranium, as in hydrocephalus or intracranial space-occupying lesion, lumbar puncture should NEVER be performed; withdrawal of fluid from the vertebral canal allows the high pressure in the ventricles to cause sudden expansion, driving the forebrain down through the tentorial notch (see 'tentorial herniation' above), and/or the brainstem and cerebellum down through the foramen magnum towards the region of lowered pressure, bringing about (frequently fatal) compression of the medulla oblongata ('coning'). For practical purposes, lumbar puncture should never be performed whenever there is ophthalmoscopic evidence of papilloedema.

# CHAPTER 6
# CEREBRAL LOCALIZATION: SPEECH AND VISUAL PATHWAYS

A rapidly-developing SOL in the supratentorial region will produce drowsiness followed by coma, probably with extensor plantar responses. Fixed dilated pupils are a very serious feature (see 'tentorial herniation', Chapter 5). If however, third nerve palsy occurs unilaterally in a case of suspected subarachnoid haemorrhage, it may indicate the side and site of the lesion on the circle of Willis.

More slowly-developing lesions, however, declare themselves less dramatically. There are two ways in which the site of a pathological process in the supratentorial region may be localized. First, it may cause dysfunction in the area in which it arises (Fig. 14); and secondly it may interfere with the visual system, which runs from front to back of the supratentorial fossae (Fig. 15).

A lesion on or near the cerebral cortex, may cause Jacksonian epilepsy—a fit which starts focally in the affected area of cortex and spreads to become generalized. Such fits may begin in part of the motor area, (e.g. by trembling of the contralateral hand), in the somatic sensory area, beginning by localized paraesthesiae, in the visual area by flashing lights in parts of the visual field, and so on. Fits having their seat in most of the non-primary cortex, however, have no localizing signs (except sometimes of side) in most instances. An exception must be made for temporal lobe epilepsy, which involves the oldest and newest parts of the cerebral

75

cortex. From the archicortex of the hippocampal gyrus and uncus may arise uncinate fits, which take the form of (usually unpleasant) olfactory hallucinations; while the temporal association neocortex (Fig. 14) gives rise to complex, multi-sensorial, integrated hallucinations, sometimes with displacement in time, which may give them a 'déjà vu' character.

Another complex 'association' area is in the frontal lobe rostral to the motor-co-ordination ('premotor') areas; lesions here are often marked by intellectual deterioration. But like the temporal lobe, in addition to this 'higher' function, the (pre-) frontal region also has a supposedly more primitive function concerned with personality (affect), due to its connections with the hypothalamus. Thus lesions can cause personality change, usually in the direction of disinhibition. Intellectual deterioration and personality change may occur together or separately. In cases where personality change is the dominating symptom, it is important to exclude organic diseases before attributing it to 'psychological' factors.

Any of the areas from which focal epilepsy may originate can also show more permanent, and obviously sometimes progressive, dysfunction. Such disorders affecting the primary motor and sensory (except auditory, because of bilateral representation) cortices can be readily understood from what has been said in earlier chapters, plus a simple knowledge of the anatomy and physiology of such areas (*IAPNS*, Chapters 10 and 13). But a lesion producing functional deficit in the cognitive association areas (*IAPNS*, Chapter 12) bordering the primary cortices can also be recognized, because they produce an appropriate form of *agnosia*. Thus for example, a lesion in parietal cortical areas 5 or 7, just behind the postcentral gyrus may, without interfering with somatic sensation as such, produce *astereognosis*, such that the subject is unable to recognize simple objects placed in the hand (with the eyes closed) or letters or numbers drawn on the skin (agraphaesthesia *or* dysgraphaesthesia). Similarly, when the visual association cortex of areas 18 and 19 is affected, there may be an inability visually to recognize objects in the affected (contralateral) hemifield—visual agnosia. A minimal degree of agnosia, due to lesions in these cognitive association areas, is seen in sensory inattention, sometimes called 'sensory extinction'. In such cases, the subject will be aware of touch, or movement in the visual hemifield, on each side when the stimuli are presented separately; but when bilateral stimuli are presented simultaneously, the patient will ignore the stimulus coming to the affected side of the brain.

It is necessary at this juncture to put in a word of warning: most patients are very eager to 'help the doctor', so if suffering from astereognosis or visual agnosia they have a tendency to say anything that comes into their heads when tested, rather than to say 'I don't recognise the object'. This has resulted in the symptom being called, in some circles, 'nominal aphasia' or 'nominal dysphasia', which naturally leads the unsuspecting student to think it is a disorder of speech, when in fact it is nothing of the sort. True disorders of speech are of localizing value, but this involves a preliminary discussion of so-called hemispheric dominance.

## HEMISPHERIC DOMINANCE AND SPEECH FUNCTION

Except in occupational circumstances leading to asymmetrical muscular development, ordinary clinical testing for power does not reveal any difference between the two upper limbs even in a strongly right- or left-handed subject. However, when a scientifically repeatable 'skilled' task is repetitively performed with both upper limbs one after the other, electromyography shows that on the dominant-side contraction of the agonist muscle(s) is accompanied by a very precisely synchronized, orderly, and repeatable activity of synergist muscles, while in the other limb the synergistic activity is absent or poorly co-ordinated, and often shows a different pattern each time the movement is performed. Such muscular activity implies that the motor and motor association (vide infra) cortex in the dominant hemisphere is much more precisely organized in a functional sense than on the non-dominant side; this, it may be argued, seems to have been unconsciously perceived by those linguistic culture-groups which use the same word for 'left' and 'clumsy' or at least 'bad right-sidedness' as in our own word 'maladroit', borrowed from French though it is.

It may easily be imagined that the muscular movements required in order to produce speech with all its subtleties require at least as high a degree of motor organization as do skilled movements of the hand; and that therefore the motor cortex which controls the dominant hand also controls the movements concerned with speech. The fact that this is not always the case, for example in born left-handers who have been successfully trained as right-handers, probably shows that speech demands even greater motor co-ordination than do most hand-movements.

The centre for the motor organization of speech (Broca's area) lies in that part of the premotor area which lies just in front of the primary motor area representation of the vocal (in the widest sense) musculature in the dominant hemisphere (Fig. 14). This premotor area is in fact a motor association area in which at more dorsal levels are represented co-ordination of eye (vide infra) and hand movements. A lesion of Broca's area gives rise to the condition of motor aphasia, in which understanding of the spoken or written word, or the ability to write, may be relatively unimpaired.

Recent work on the functional asymmetry of the two cerebral hemispheres in man has tended, in rather gross and imprecise terms, to label the dominant hemisphere as logical or rational and the other as emotional or poetical. In view of this, it is extremely interesting to note that some patients

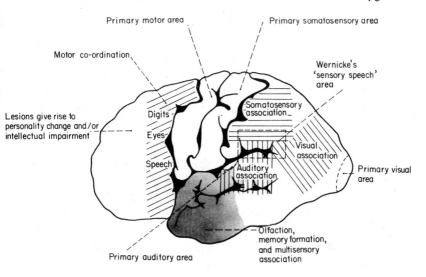

Fig. 14. Diagram of the lateral surface of the left cerebral hemisphere to show functional areas. See text for explanation of syndromes arising from dysfunction of individual areas.

with motor aphasia, unable to speak a sentence, are capable of swearing and singing—both of which may be regarded as emotional rather than rational activities.

Since the primary sensory areas are bordered by their specific cognitive association areas, it is evident that the somatic, visual, and auditory cognitive association areas meet approximately in the region where the lateral fissure turns dorsally towards its occipital end (Fig. 14). It seems that in this junctional region, the blood supply is not separate for each functional area, so that it is extremely rare to encounter a lesion involving only one of them. In any event, the whole region, under the title of Wernicke's area, is concerned with understanding of the spoken and written word so that lesions lead to failure of these functions—word deafness or word blindness (alexia). This region is also connected with the motor speech area by corticocortical association fibres, such as the superior longitudinal and frontooccipital fasciculi, so that lesions in it may also affect verbal expression—either by total or partial aphasia, or unintelligible jargon speech; it should be mentioned that true nominal aphasia (vide supra) can be seen as a result of a lesion in the cortical areas concerned with speech.

## CORTICAL CONTROL OF EYE MOVEMENTS

A fairly close parallel can be drawn between the speech areas and those responsible for eye movements—except that the latter are bilaterally represented, and ipsilateral cortico-cortical connections perhaps less important.

The frontal eye field is in the same premotor area as the motor speech area (Fig. 14), but at a higher (i.e. more dorsal) level—because the face is represented the right way up in the motor and motor association cortex. Stimulation of the frontal eye field by an electrode or by an epileptic discharge causes conjugate deviation of the eyes to the contralateral side, i.e. to the side from which visual impulses come into the stimulated hemisphere. By the same token, a destructive lesion of the frontal eye field makes the patient incapable of voluntarily directing the gaze to the contralateral side; but the eyes will still turn to the contralateral side when following a slowly moving object which has been fixated when still directly in front of the eyes. This serves to differentiate a lesion of the frontal eye field from one in the lower brainstem involving the medial longitudinal fasciculus in the region of the abducent nucleus, for in the latter case conjugate lateral gaze (to the side of the lesion) is impossible either voluntarily or reflexly.

Eye movements of two sorts are controlled from the occipital cortex—the active region in this instance involving not only the visual association areas (18 and 19) but also the primary visual cortex (area 17). In the normal, under control of the occipital cortex of both sides working together, the eyes (i) move to follow an object which has been visually fixed, and (ii) accommodate to focus the fixed object. These are usually called the fixation and accommodaton reflexes, but in fact they are almost inextricably linked. The human eyes automatically fix on something, and the normal fixation reflex is responsible for the normal phenomenon of opto-kinetic nystagmus, which can be seen for example in someone who is looking out of the window of a moving train.

The fixation and accommodation reflexes are not dependent, like speech functions, on corticocortical connections, but on direct corticotectal connections. Stimulation of the occipital cortex, as of the frontal eye field, causes the eyes to deviate conjugately towards the side from which the stimulated cortex receives its light, i.e. to the contralateral side. Unilateral lesions in the area, in the rare instances that they do not also interfere with visual function, cause loss of both fixation and accommodation in the affected visual hemifield, so that vision is described as blurred, especially if the subject, or the object being looked at, is moving. There is no inability to move the eyes voluntarily in any direction in such cases.

## THE VISUAL SYSTEM (Fig. 15)

Because it is large (each human optic nerve and tract consists of about a million fibres), because it extends from the front to the back of the supratentorial region, and because both subject and examiner are highly aware of it, the visual system has an enormous value in the localization of cerebral lesions.

The optic nerve has already been dealt with (Chapter 1). The manner of crossing of optic fibres (from the nasal halves of the retinae only) is so well-known as to need no further reiteration. The visual pathway is equally precisely organized in the superoinferior direction; retinal efferents maintain these relative positions throughout. Each eye is essentially a pinhole camera, in which light rays coming from different

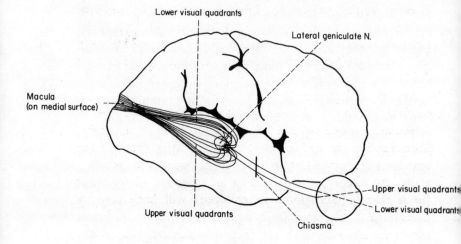

FIG. 15. The visual system projected onto the lateral surface of the cerebral hemisphere (after Cushing).

directions cross at the pupil; given this, the organisation of the visual pathways is such that all light coming from the left passes into the right optic tract (and vice versa), while light coming from above activates fibres in the ventral (inferior) part of both visual pathways, and vice versa. It should be noted that *visual signs and symptoms are always spoken of in terms of the direction from which light comes*, and not in terms of the part of the retina illuminated or fibres activated; thus, for example, the deficit resulting from failure to appreciate light (from the left) falling on the nasal half of the left retina and the temporal half of the right retina (which should be due to a lesion in the post-decussational visual pathway on the right) is spoken of as a left homonymous hemianopia.

It must be further remembered that the afferent fibres responsible for pupillary changes (light and accommodation reflexes) are retino-tectal; they are apparently bilaterally distributed from each eye. Unlike visuosensory fibres, they do not relay in the lateral geniculate nucleus, but pass directly to the tectum in the brachium of the superior colliculus, so that beyond (behind) the lateral geniculate the visuosensory and pupillary reflex fibres are anatomically separated, the former travelling in the optic radiation and the latter in the brachium.

Armed with this information (provided he/she has it correctly) even the tyro can localize a very large number of intracranial lesions with a considerable degree of accuracy. Consider first the *optic chiasma*. This is related above to the anterior communicating artery and below to the pituitary gland. An aneurysm of the former or a tumour of the latter (or a craniopharyngioma in children) will both cause a bitemporal hemianopia if they are exactly in the midline and catch the decussating fibres from the nasal halves of the retinae; but pressure from above will first affect vision in the inferior temporal quadrant of the visual field and pressure from below vision in the superior temporal quadrant. All of the conditions mentioned are often, in fact, slightly away from the midline, in which case they tend to affect vision in one eye (i.e. by compressing the optic nerve) first, but will still affect the inferior or superior halves of the fields according to their position.

A lesion in the optic tract between the chiasma and the lateral geniculate produces a homonymous hemianopia in the contralateral visual field, together with a loss of the light reflex provided that only the affected parts of the retinae are illuminated, which in practice is an exceedingly difficult thing to do. It must be remembered that normally the head and eyes are turned so as to focus any fixated object on the macula; for this reason, to the great surprise of both patient and examiner, homonymous hemianopia may go unnoticed until the visual fields are tested by confrontation or perimetry.

Should the optic radiation be affected in its entirety homonymous hemianopia also results; but with sparing of the light reflex since retinotectal fibres separate from the visual pathway behind the lateral geniculate. However, the optic radiation is much more spread out than is the tract, so that partial field defects are much commoner in post-geniculate than in pregeniculate lesions; for example, a temporal lobe tumour may produce an upper quadrantic defect in the contralateral half of the visual field.

The visual cortex is more often affected by vascular lesions involving the posterior cerebral artery than by space-occupying lesions. To repeat, a total lesion will produce homonymous hemianopia; but the representation of the retinae on the cortex should be considered. The macula is represented (bilaterally) at the occipital pole, so that a small unilateral lesion here may produce no observable field defect, though fixation and accommodation may be affected. Peripheral vision is represented further forwards.

A lesion between the occipital cortex and the tectum may affect the pupillary accommodation reflex while the light reflex remains normal. This however is even rarer than the famous 'Argyll Robertson pupil' in which a pupil of irregular outline reacts to accommodation but not to light. It is believed to be due to a lesion (usually syphilitic) of the pretectal region of the midbrain.

Midbrain lesions are also responsible for certain disorders of ocular movement. Irritative lesions of the rostral tectum are believed to be responsible for oculogyric crises, in which the eyes involuntarily deviate upwards, while compressive lesions in the same region (e.g. from bilateral chronic sub-dural haematomata or a tumour in the pineal region) cause paralysis of upward gaze. If the compression spreads further back, downward gaze will also be affected.

Intracranial space-occupying lesions produce a deformation of the brain. While this obviously occurs at the site of the SOL, it may also occur at a distance, due to displacement. Tentorial herniation has already been mentioned (Chapter 5,) but displacement of this type is likely in the first instance to affect those cranial nerves which have the longest course and the most delicate structure, i.e. the sixth and fourth. The midbrain may be twisted, or compressed against the edges of the tentorial notch. According to the direction of displacement, various disorders arise (see Chapter 5) one of which may be ipsilateral hemiparesis; or tectal lesions, as described above, may also be seen.

All the above are false localizing signs; they may of course co-exist with true localizing signs, rendering diagnosis of the primary lesion site extremely difficult. Recourse to such procedures as brain scan, angiography to reveal displacement of vessels or abnormal circulation, ventriculography, or computerized tomography will be necessary in order to decide what exactly is amiss.

# CHAPTER 7
# PAIN

Pain from the skin is divisible into two components: first, pricking, or fast pain, which is rapidly conducted to consciousness, well localized, and does not outlast the application of the provoking stimulus; and second or slow pain which takes an appreciable time to reach consciousness from the extremities, is poorly localized, and outlasts the application of the provoking stimulus.

Pricking sensation, although called first pain, is not regarded as painful by most subjects. It is conveyed by impulses in high-threshold mechanoreceptor A$\delta$ fibres in the tegument (skin, cornea, teeth), which on reaching the spinal cord or brainstem bring about a withdrawal (flexion) reflex when activated. This is in the first instance a segmental reflex, resulting only in withdrawal of the stimulated part; but impulses may also travel up to a centre in the medullary reticular formation and down again to lower motor neurones in many segments, resulting in withdrawal of the whole organism (spinobulbospinal reflex). The biological purpose of the withdrawal reflex is to protect the organism against potential damage.

Second or true pain is associated with repetitive stimulation of C-fibre polymodal nociceptors, so called because they can be activated by mechanical, thermal, or chemical stimulation; the common element in all these is probably tissue damage. Polymodal nociceptors are found not only in the tegument, but also in the deep tissues including the viscera. When impulses from these C fibres, unaccompanied by activity in Aδ fibres, reach the spinal cord or brainstem, they cause reflex tonic rigidity in the striated musculature supplied from the same segment, as can be seen in the guarding of acute appendicitis or the spasm surrounding a dislocation or fracture. The biological purpose of this reflex is to rest the affected part, allowing the maximal opportunity for 'natural' cure.

Pricking sensation reaches consciousness by travelling in neospinothalamic or trigeminothalamic fibres to the ventro-posterior thalamic nucleus and thence to the postcentral gyrus (*IAPNS*, Chapter 10), whereas impulses generated by true pain travel not only by this route, but also by spino-reticular fibres (also in the anterolateral quadrant of the spinal white matter) to the ascending reticular formation of the brainstem, whence they are distributed to widespread diencephalic areas and so to virtually the whole cortex (*IAPNS*, Chapter 11).

The information carried in the extralemniscal fibres of the anterolateral quadrant of the spinal cord is consciously interpreted as belonging to a whole range of ill-defined sensory experiences—varying from itch to agony—which are sometimes grouped under the heading of 'protopathic sensa-tion'. Present-day theories suggest that the conscious sensory quality resulting from impulse traffic passing up the antero-lateral column through the reticular formation to dien-cephalon and cortex is quantity-dependent; that is to say that slight activation may be interpreted as itch while intense activation is translated as pain.

There are a number of inhibitory control mechanisms acting on this system, as there are on all ascending sensory systems. The first acts at segmental level, and is known as the 'gate control' mechanism, because it is thought to open or (partially) close a 'gate' which controls the amount of peripherally-generated information passing up the antero-

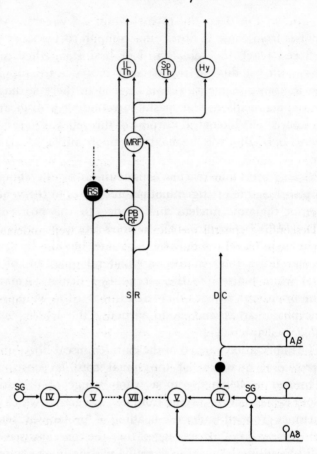

FIG. 16. Connections of the extralemniscal components of the antero-lateral system. SG, IV, V, and VII are Rexed laminae of the spinal grey matter. Spinoreticular fibres (SR) take off from lamina VIII (and VIII, not shown) to reach mainly the pontobulbar reticular formation (PBRF) and to a lesser extent the midbrain reticular formation (MRF). Ascending reticular projections reach the intralaminar (ILTh) and specific (SpTh) thalamic nuclei and hypothalamus (Hy), and thence most regions of the cortex. The SR system is activated by convergence from A$\delta$ and C peripheral afferents, but this can be partly blocked through the activation of the segmental inhibitory interneurone (black) by activation of the large (A$\beta$) primary afferent, either orthodromically in the periphery or antidromically from the dorsal columns (DC). The descending inhibitory

lateral columns (Fig. 16). Collaterals of the large (A$\beta$) low-threshold mechanoreceptor primary afferents which form the dorsal columns are believed to activate inhibitory interneurones at segmental entry level, which in their turn act on neurones in the spinal grey chain leading to cells whose axons forms the anterolateral columns. Thus activation of low-threshold mechanoreceptors in the periphery will reduce the amount of traffic passing up the anterolateral columns; a practical application of this is seen in the universal human habit of lightly rubbing the skin over a painful area, 'to make it better' as children say after being hurt.

Descending control mechanisms are less well understood. They are evidently under eventual cortical control, like all others. As at present known, lower parts of this system (Fig. 16) consist of midbrain reticular (periaqueductal) neurones which probably excite inhibitory reticulospinal cells in the medulla oblongata; the axons of the latter act on spinal neurones which form part of the chain giving rise to ascending anterolateral fibres. The cells in this descending inhibitory chain are believed to be activated by a naturally-occurring peptide transmitter, enkephalin, whose actions in this respect are mimicked by morphine.

Although neither the site nor the mechanism of the cortical control of these descending inhibitory pathways is known, they are of great importance. For example, it is well known that soldiers on the battlefield or sportsmen in the midst of an exciting game are frequently unaware of sustaining an injury which in other circumstances would be extremely painful. Similarly, the practitioners of certain

reticulospinal system (RS) can be activated either from above by the descending enkephalinergic fibres (dotted arrow), or by collaterals from neighbouring excitatory ascending reticular cells (PBRF). Note that the two kinds of inhibition are effected on different laminae in the spinal grey matter.

mystery cults, such as Indian fakirs, are apparently able to 'switch off' conscious pain sensation, as are some devout Western political or religious believers when subjected to torture. Unfortunately these people do not know how they do it, so that it is not at present possible to exploit the mechanism for medical purposes. It is important, however, to appreciate that all these subjects are genuinely unaware of the painful quality of noxious stimuli—they do not just grin and bear it.

It may be appropriate at this point to mention hypnosis, which may activate the same unknown mechanisms. In the hands of expert medical hypnotists, it has been found that pain sensation caused by organic changes can be suppressed while the patient is 'under the influence'; while pain of psychogenic origin is not influenced by hypnosis. This distinction in effect is said to be so clear that hypnosis may be used as a differential diagnostic procedure to determine whether a given pain is of organic or psychogenic origin. It should be added parenthetically that psychogenic pain hurts the patient as much as does organic; it should not be dismissed, but referred for expert psychiatric treatment.

In clinical practice, it is regrettably common to determine whether a patient can distinguish the sharp from the blunt end of a pin, and if not, to say that there is a loss or diminution of 'pain sensation'. It cannot be strongly enough emphasized that what is being tested by this procedure is pricking sensation, abnormalities of which alone virtually never bring patients to seek medical advice, and whose anatomical pathways are separate from those of true pain above the spinal cord.

True pain sensation is more difficult and time-consuming to test. If the lower extremity is involved, it may be done by pinching the Achilles tendon—but the lower extremity is not always necessarily implicated. Perhaps the most satisfactory way to test true pain sensation in the limbs is by inducing muscle ischaemia. This is done by inflating a sphygmomanometer cuff around the limb to above systolic pressure and instructing the patient to make alternating movements, such as clenching and unclenching the hand, or rising onto the toes, to a metronome or loudly-ticking clock. The test should be applied simultaneously to affected and unaffected limbs; the measure is expressed as the length of time required to induce muscle pain in the control and affected limbs. If there is no pain on the affected side five minutes after it occurs on the control side, the test may be regarded as positive and discontinued. A qualitative, but not quantitative, test for the presence or absence of true pain can be quickly carried out by applying potassium chloride solution to a discontinuity, such as a graze, in the skin. Normally this chemogenic sensation, induced by rubbing salt into a wound, is agonizing, as the putative practitioner can and should find out for himself; but it can be quickly got rid of by running water onto the site of application.

## DISORDERS OF PAIN SENSATION

First or pricking pain acts as a warning against impending damage, and second or real pain, when appearing spontaneously, is usually a signal of disease which ought to be attended to. Thus total or partial loss of either type of sensation may be dangerous. This can be seen in the rare cases of congenital absence of pain sensation; the subjects usually die at a relatively early age from unsuspected disease. The few pathological reports available on such cases suggest that there is an absence of small peripheral fibres and/or of the substantia gelatinosa of the spinal grey matter and descending trigeminal nucleus in which these fibres relay.

In disease, the two forms of pain may be interfered with, together or separately, at any point between the periphery and the forebrain. Some knowledge of physiological mechanisms and anatomical pathways allows a differential diagnosis to be made.

Peripherally, small fibres may be specifically attacked, leading to loss of pain sensation in the affected area. Leprosy, happily a disappearing disease, is an example of this. More frequently encountered is tabes dorsalis, a form of tertiary syphilis which attacks the dorsal columns of the spinal cord (leading to partial loss of mechanoreceptive functions) and the dorsal roots of spinal nerves, where the smallest fibres appear to be selected, particularly (though for unknown reasons) those coming from joints. Sufferers from the disease usually exhibit painless hyperextension or hyperflexion of joints in the affected region (usually the lower limbs), and may have painless swelling and destruction of the joints (Charcot's joints) due to unfelt insult to the joint surfaces. There is an interesting reaction to scratching or pinching the skin of the extremity: a delayed and slow flexion (withdrawal) reflex. This is usually attributed to delayed conduction through the affected dorsal roots.

Equal and opposite, as it were, to these peripheral nerve afflictions in which painful sensation is lost or diminished are the conditions in which pain is intensified. Since they are all believed to be due to functional or anatomical interference with large low-threshold mechanoreceptive fibres, they are explained by the absence of 'gate control', i.e. when impulses from large fibres fail to reach the spinal cord, they obviously cannot activate the inhibitory interneurones at segmental entry level, so that input from small fibres is not partially suppressed as would normally be the case, and painful sensation is enhanced. Such a mechanism may be responsible for the 'lightning pains' and tabetic crises which can occur in tabes dorsalis, the former usually being referred to long bones and the latter to abdominal viscera.

However, the simplest illustration of large fibre dysfunction is in the hyperalgesia of skin which is being re-innervated by regenerating fibres following traumatic interruption of a cutaneous nerve branch. Nerve injury is of course followed immediately by total anaesthesia in the appropriate area of skin. But when the nerve begins to regenerate, it has been shown that small fibres grow faster than large ones, so that a phase occurs when the affected area of skin is re-innervated by small, but not by large, fibres. It is at this stage that an appropriate stimulus will induce a more intensely painful sensation than when applied to normal skin. Later, when the regeneration of large fibres is complete, the hyperalgesia disappears.

Since large fibres are more susceptible than small to ischaemia (see Chapter 1), it is possible that pains such as that of sciatica due to herniation of an inter-vertebral disc, or that felt in the upper extremity in the brachial plexus and carpal tunnel syndromes, may be caused by mechanical interference with the blood supply to nerve trunks, resulting in functional inactivation of the larger fibres. In all these conditions there is frequently loss or diminution of low-threshold mechanoreceptive sensation and muscle weakness, signifying loss of function in large peripheral fibres.

An irreversible change may occur in post-herpetic neuralgia. In this virus disease, which occurs most frequently in the first division of the trigeminal nerve and in the intercostal nerves, the cell bodies of large afferent fibres are affected and may be destroyed in the trigeminal or dorsal root ganglia (compare the destruction of lower motor neurone cell bodies by poliomyelitis virus). Stimulation of the receptors activating the remaining small fibres results in intense, often apparently spontaneous, pain.

Following partial lesions, particularly to nerve trunks in the upper limb, apparently spontaneous intense burning pains may develop in the condition known as *causalgia*. This differs from post-herpetic neuralgia chiefly in that, because the lesion occurs below the level of union of dorsal and ventral roots, there is evidence of activity in (unmyelinated) autonomic efferent fibres. Otherwise, it is also believed to be due to failure of 'gate control'.

Within the central nervous system, there is only one common condition in which the pathological process is suspected as possibly having its seat at the level of the first central synapse at root entry level. This is *trigeminal neuralgia*, which commonly occurs idiopathically in elderly subjects and is characterized by episodes of shooting pain in the distribution of one or more divisions of the trigeminal nerve, or much more rarely in the pharyngeal distribution of the ninth nerve.

Because attacks may be triggered by even a low-intensity stimulus in the area supplied by the affected nerve, a peripheral cause has been intensively sought, but not found; in contradistinction to the true peripheral affections described above, there is no abnormality of any somatosensory modality between attacks. The most favoured (but still unproven) explanation at the present time is an epileptiform discharge in the descending trigeminal nucleus, in which the small somatic afferent fibres of the trigeminal and glossopharyngeal nerves terminate. Triggering by a low-intensity peripheral stimulus is explained on this hypothesis by the fact that large low-threshold fibres also have a branch ending in the same nucleus, and it is supposed that its hyperexcitable cells are provoked to epileptic-type discharge by an afferent excitation. The strongest evidence for the epileptiform nature of trigeminal neuralgia is derived from the fact that many cases can be controlled by the administration of an anti-epileptic drug, Carbamazepine,

In the spinal cord, it is evident that any lesion interrupting the spinoreticular and neospinothalamic pathways in the anterolateral quadrant of the white matter will abolish, contralaterally, the ability to feel either type of pain (see Fig. 6); indeed, it was from the careful study a well-circumscribed tuberculoma in the anterolateral white column that present knowledge of its function was established at the beginning of the present century. In human pathology, the most commonly-occurring such condition is syringomyelia (and the anatomically similar haematomyelia), which for practical purposes may be regarded as a cavity in the cord spreading anterolaterally from the central canal. While the disease has additional effects on lower motor neurones and upper motor neurones, the most striking symptoms in the present context are analgesia and thermanaesthesia covering the contralateral half of the body from about four to six segments below the highest part of the lesion. Patients with this disease frequently present on account of painless infected wounds in which the original trauma went unnoticed. On somatosensory testing, there is a level below which thermal, pricking, and truly painful stimuli are not felt, except for their essential tactile element, while mechanoreceptive functions are unimpaired; this phenomenon is known as 'dissociated sensory loss'.

At higher levels of the neuraxis, it is unusual to find lesions which produce pure deficits of painful sensation. There are well-defined syndromes resulting from lesions in the brainstem and diencephalon which demonstrate the incompleteness of our knowledge of the anatomical and physiological mechanisms underlying painful sensation, and present a challenge to the investigator.

For example, thrombosis of the posterior inferior cerebellar artery (Fig. 11) or its medullary branches produces necrosis of the lateral part of the lower medulla oblongata, which contains the upward continuation of the ascending antero-lateral column of the spinal cord. Such a lesion, however, may sometimes produce not only analgesia and thermanaesthesia in the contralateral half of the body, but also spontaneous pain referred to the analgesic portion of the body—a true, and highly distressing, anaesthesia dolorosa. The usual explanation is that the anterolateral ascending fibres are irritated, but this does not stand up to critical examination. It is more likely that in those cases of posterior inferior cerebellar artery syndrome in which spontaneous pain occurs, there is interference with the descending inhibitory reticulospinal system referred to at the beginning of the chapter.

The thalamic syndrome occurs when the ventroposterior nucleus of the thalamus is destroyed almost invariably by arterial thrombosis. Since this nucleus is the relay to the cortex of the medial lemniscus, the neospinothalamic tract, and their trigeminal homologues, there results a loss of mechanoreceptive and thermoreceptive sensation in the opposite half of the body and face, accompanied by spontaneous pain in the anaesthetic area. The very existence of such a syndrome implies that there must be a further 'gating' mechanism at thalamic level, though its nature is not at present understood. The lateral medullary syndrome is often confused with, and misdiagnosed as, thalamic syndrome; but the (usual) preservation of mechanoreceptive function in the former should enable a distinction to be made.

The postcentral gyrus or the thalamocortical projections to it are sometimes affected by a vascular or neoplastic lesion, which may be small enough to cause loss of conscious somatic sensation in only part of the body. Particularly in lesions deep to the cortical surface, it is not uncommon to observe loss of pinprick sensation and thermanaesthesia, together of course with loss of low-threshold mechanoreceptive sensation, but with preservation of true pain. Such a syndrome serves as a reminder that pricking (first pain) and thermal sensations are caused by impulses travelling up the neospinothalamic tract and relayed to the postcentral cortex through the ventroposterior thalamic nucleus, while impulses interpreted as true pain reach more widespread areas of cortex through a variety of other diencephalic relays.

## TREATMENT OF PAIN AS A SYMPTOM

Although both pricking and true pain serve a useful biological purpose, and should be relieved by successful treatment of the causative disease, there are instances in which either the disease itself cannot be alleviated (e.g. widespread malignant disease) or in which a permanent change is caused by the disease, resulting in continued, sometimes continuous, and biologically useless true pain. Continuous pain is degrading, distressing, and greatly detracts from human dignity, and so should be symptomatically treated. Since pain itself is not a disease, and its treatment throws considerable light on its mechanisms, some methods of pain relief will be discussed here in terms of their anatomy and physiology.

*Local anaesthesia* may be used to block input from a peripheral site which is causing pain. Repeated injections may succeed in permanently abolishing pain sensation. The fact that this therapeutic measure is so frequently successful has lead to the hypothesis that long-term afferent bombardment may sensitize central cells transsynaptically—an extension of the phenomenon of 'windup', whereby the response of central cells to C fibre input increases successively. It may be that the periods of rest for central cells induced by peripheral anaesthesia allows them to recuperate and lose their hypersensitivity.

It will be recalled that many afferents from abdominothoracic viscera pass through autonomic ganglia. Transient inactivation by local anaesthetics or permanent inactivation by injection of alcohol or phenol have an excellent record as pain-relieving procedures in cases of visceral pain. Recent observations suggest that some C fibres enter the spinal cord in ventral roots, which is perhaps one reason why peripheral autonomic block is often more successful than dorsal rhizotomy.

*Dorsal rhizotomy* obviously abolishes all afferent input through the sectioned root. It is rather a heroic measure to undertake, since not only are all the represented somato-sensory submodalities eliminated, but also the stretch receptor input essential for muscle control. Moreover, the smaller fibres in the dorsal roots, on entry into the spinal cord, extend up and down a surprisingly large number of segments by collateral branching. Thus there is extensive overlap, and it often proves necessary to cut a large number of roots in order to abolish pain in quite a small area, while at the same time abolishing everything else over a wide area. This is the main reason why surgical rhizotomy, with one exception to be mentioned below, is now not very frequently undertaken. Another reason is that the pain of a number of conditions with peripheral pathology, such as post-herpetic neuralgia, is not usually abolished by rhizotomy. This must mean either that such conditions have an unknown central component in their pathology, *or* that following prolonged pathological bombardment, central neurones become super-sensitive or develop autonomous discharge patterns. The second possibility receives considerable support from the ineffectiveness of rhizotomy for phantom limb pain following amputation, where no possibility of central pathology arises.

Widespread rhizotomy would be more acceptable if only the small fibres in the dorsal roots were destroyed, and this is the rationale of chemical rhizotomy. In this procedure, a chemical substance, usually phenol in low concentration, is injected intrathecally and manoeuvred into the little conical pockets of the subarachnoid space which mark the points of entry of the dorsal roots. Because small fibres are unprotected by myelin, or have only a little, they are more susceptible to irreversible or reversible chemical damage (*cf.* the effect of procaine on dental nerves).

The one situation in which rhizotomy is highly effective is the sensory root of the trigeminal nerve, where it can be carried out by open surgery or by injection of alcohol into the Gasserian ganglion; recently, techniques for the selective destruction of small trigeminal root fibres by radiofrequency lesions have become available. Whether all fibres or only small fibres are destroyed, the corneal reflex is abolished, which means that the eye must be carefully protected after operation. Trigeminal root section is eminently successful in abolishing trigeminal neuralgia (but not post-herpetic neuralgia in the trigeminal distribution). This lends credence to the 'epilepsy' theory of idiopathic trigeminal neuralgia, for it eliminates afferent bombardment of the trigeminal nuclei.

The most universally effective manoeuvre for pain relief is *anterolateral cordotomy*, which may be performed either by open surgery or by thermocoagulation through a percutaneously inserted electrode. Because such a procedure destroys both neospinothalamic and spinoreticular fibres in the one place where they run together, both first and second pain (as well as thermal sensation) are totally abolished on the contralateral side of the body up to a level from four to six segments below the level of operation, with preservation of low-threshold mechanoreceptive sensation. Furthermore, it is possible to perform the operation bilaterally, even at cervical level, provided the two procedures are separated by a suitable lapse of time.

Anterolateral cordotomy is the operation of choice in patients with a limited expectation of life, such as those with malignant disease. However, in cases of long survival, there is a tendency for pain sensation to return after an interval of nine to eighteen months. It is not known at present whether this is due to the opening up of 'alternative pathways', whatever they are (though this is the classical explanation), or the reoccupation of vacated synaptic sites in the brainstem by collateral sprouting of intact spinoreticular fibres.

Again, *destructive surgical intervention in the intralaminar thalamus*, on the grounds that it is the chief thalamic end-situation for ascending reticular projections, usually has a very short-lived effect (one to three months). This is probably because ascending reticular fibres are widely distributed to other areas of the thalamus and hypothalamus. An exception may be made for thalamotomy in the case of oro-facial pain, because in this instance a single lesion can destroy the intralaminar nuclei and the adjacent medial ventroposterior nucleus, which is the specific somatosensory relay for the head and face.

By the same token, *alcohol injection into the pituitary fossa* which may destroy part of the hypothalamus as well as the hypophysis, has been found to be effective, bilaterally for the control of pain from malignant disease.

Finally among destructive procedures, bilateral severance of the projections from the dorsomedial thalamic nucleus to the prefrontal cortex (*frontal lobotomy*) has been found to abolish the affective component of pain, so that such patients say they feel pain but do not care about it any more. The operation is only undertaken in extreme cases because of its undesirable effects on personality and vegetative functions; but it demonstrates not only the widespread (and bilateral) cortical regions involved in the normal appreciation of pain, but the exceedingly complex and diverse mechanisms which must be concerned.

The non-destructive treatment of pain offers some fascinating insights. The ill-understood cortical control of descending inhibitory mechanisms was illustrated by some naturally-occurring examples at the beginning of this chapter. It is of considerable interest that pain of organic origin can be abolished by hypnosis, pain sensation being absent so long as the patient is under the spell. Medical hypnotists use the technique as a diagnostic test, since although pain of organic origin can be suppressed, psychogenic pain is unaffected by hypnosis.

It has been mentioned above that the downwardly-projecting reticular neurones in the meso-diencephalic periaqueductal region, whose axons terminate on inhibitory reticulospinal neurones in the lower brainstem, work by a

naturally-occurring morphinomimetic polypeptide, enkephalin. It is at this level that morphine and its analogues
act. Now that the composition of enkephalin is known, it is
to be hoped that drugs having the pain-suppressing effect of
morphine but without its undesirable side-effects may become
available. In the meanwhile, some neurosurgeons have
claimed success for the stimulation of the periaqueductal-
periventricular grey matter by an implanted electrode; such
stimulation had previously been shown to reduce the
reaction to noxious stimulation in experimental animals.

Those medullary reticulospinal cells which give rise to
descending inhibitory axons may be implicated in the rather
rare but spectacular instances when heterosegmentally-
applied acupuncture is successful in abolishing pain, since
this particular region of the reticular formation has been
found to be excited by pricking-type peripheral stimuli at
rates not exceeding 3 per second.

Stimulation therapy has found its most successful application so far in exploitation of the (modified) 'gate control'
theory. Large low-threshold primary afferent fibres may be
stimulated by low-intensity high-frequency electrical currents
either transcutaneously by means of surface electrodes, or
by an electrode implanted on a peripheral nerve, or antidromically by an electrode implanted over the dorsal
columns. In all of these cases, (Fig. 16), such stimulation
presumably activates, by segmental collaterals, inhibitory
interneurones which act on cells of origin of anterolateral
fibres.

Just as there are unsolved mysteries in the production of
pain and in the recovery of pain sensation after cordotomy,
so there are in the pain-suppressing effects of stimulation.
For example, while no neurophysiological effects with
durations of more than a few thousand milliseconds have
been demonstrated in the laboratory, both electrical and
acupuncture stimulation of a few minutes' duration may
bring about relief for hours or even days. Many more

instances could be enumerated, but these will perhaps suffice to persuade the reader that the understanding of pain is only at its beginning.

# INDEX

Blindness 17
Brachium conjunctivum 60
Bradycardia 69
Brainstem 86, 87, 95, 99
  compression of 64, 69, 70
  and hypoglossal nerve 22
  lesions in 34, 43, 51, 80
  and lumbar puncture 74
  and nystagmus 15
  and paresis 33
  reticulospinal neurones in 100
  and trigeminal sensory nuclei
    19
Broca's (motor speech) area 78

Canals, semicircular 13, 14, 15,
  62
Carbamazepine 94
Causalgia 20, 93
Cavernous sinus 8, 12, 19
Cerebellum 15, 26, 36, 48, 49,
  58–64, 70, 74
Cerebrospinal fluid 66–74
Cervical rib 2, 4
Charcot's joints 92
Chiasma, optic 16, 83
Chorea 39
Choroid plexus 71, 73
Chronic bulbar palsy 4, 38
Circle of Willis 68, 75
Cisternal puncture 69
Cisterna Magna 68, 69
Clonus 27
Compression, *see also* Pressure
  intracranial *and* Space-
  occupying lesion
  of brain 67
  of brainstem 64, 69, 70
  of cerebellum 57
  of cerebral peduncle 7
  of flocculus 62
  of medulla oblongata 74

  of medullary pyramid 31
  of midbrain 85
  of nerves 2, 3, 4, 5, 12
  of optic nerve 17, 83
  in posterior fossa 14, 65
  of spinal cord 40, 41, 42, 43,
    50–51
  in subarachnoid haemorrhage
    68
  tectal 84
  of tegmentum 37
  of vestibular nuclei 63
Colliculus, superior, brachium
  of 83
Cordotomy, anterolateral 99, 101
Cornea 18
Corpus callosum 30
Corpus Striatum 26
Cortex
  cerebral 23, 40
    and alcohol 62
    and cerebellum 58
    and epilepsy 75–76
    and the eye 16
    and hydrocephalus 73
    and pain 87, 96, 100
    and paresis 33
    and tonic inhibition 36
  motor coordination 76, 78
  motor, principal 23, 29–30,
    31, 32, 34, 35, 38, 76, 78
  motor, supplementary 23, 30,
    34–35, 75
  occipital 80, 81, 84
  sensory 76, 79
  somatosensory 3, 49, 75
  speech 78–80
  visual 75, 80, 84
  visual association 77, 80
Craniopharyngioma 83
Curare 5
Cyst 67